GERD DIET COOKBOOK FOR SENIORS

The Comprehensive Guide to Healthy and Delicious Recipes to manage and reverse Acid Reflux

Cody C. Knight

HOW TO USE THIS COOKBOOK

Become familiar with GERD

Before getting into the cookbook, learn about Gastroesophageal Reflux Disease (GERD), including its symptoms, triggers, and how it affects seniors in particular. This core knowledge will enable you to make informed decisions along your journey.

Learn the Basics of the GERD Diet

Read the chapter on the diet's guidelines. Understand which foods you should avoid and which are okay to eat. Pay attention to portion amounts and eating habits that may help ease discomfort.

Plan Your Meals

Follow the sample meal plans in the guidebook for breakfast, lunch, supper, and snacks. These plans are intended to provide a foundation for preparing balanced, GERD-friendly meals. Personalize them based on your preferences and dietary requirements.

Explore Recipes

Browse through the recipe chapters, which are organized by meal type. Each meal is carefully designed to be GERD-friendly, with an emphasis on whole, minimally processed ingredients that are kind on the digestive tract. Choose meals that are appealing to you and meet your dietary requirements.

Follow Cooking directions

Carefully follow the recipes' directions. Make a note of any suggested substitutes or changes to make the food more appropriate for your needs. Experiment with different cooking methods and taste combinations to keep your meals interesting.

Monitor Your Body

As you incorporate GERD-friendly foods into your diet, pay attention to how your body reacts. Observe any changes in your symptoms and modify your diet accordingly. Keep notice of the foods that appear to cause discomfort and avoid them in the future.

Maintain Consistency

Managing GERD through food requires a long-term commitment. Maintain consistency in your food planning and cooking efforts, especially when faced with obstacles or setbacks. Remember that every nutritious meal you eat contributes to better symptom management and overall wellness.

Seek Support

If you have questions or concerns about managing GERD through food, consult healthcare specialists or support groups. They can offer vital advice and encouragement along the way.

Enjoy the benefits

Finally, enjoy the benefits of a GERD-friendly diet. Consume meals that nourish your body and promote digestive wellness. Accept the opportunity to take charge of

your health and well-being through mindful eating habits.

TABLE OF CONTENTS

INTRODUCTION

Olivia sat in her warm kitchen, marveling at the bright fruits and veggies on her countertop. It wasn't simply any random collection of veggies; each item had been meticulously chosen to fit her stringent GERD diet. Olivia's life with Gastroesophageal Reflux Disease had been a daily battle, but she had found consolation and control in her culinary choices.

Her path to treating GERD through food had not been easy. Years ago, Olivia was constantly troubled by unpleasant symptoms, including a burning sensation in her chest, a bitter taste in her mouth, and constant discomfort after meals. She visited doctors and tried various drugs, but nothing appeared to provide long-term relief. Frustrated and resolved to take matters into her own hands, Olivia conducted research and discovered the possibility of dietary changes in GERD management.

Olivia set off on a dietary transformation quest, armed with her newly acquired information. She no longer enjoyed spicy dishes, acidic fruits, and greasy pleasures. In their place, she adopted a diet high in whole grains, lean meats, and fiber-rich fruits and vegetables. It was a significant shift, but

Olivia was determined to do whatever it needed to regain control of her health and well-being.

As she methodically sliced veggies for a colorful stir-fry, Olivia thought on the wonderful changes she had noticed since starting her GERD-friendly diet. The frequent bouts of heartburn were a distant memory, replaced with a renewed sense of vitality and comfort. She no longer dreaded dinner since she knew that each dish she cooked was not only fueling her body but also nurturing her spirit.

However, Olivia's journey was not without difficulties. There were times when she wished for a slice of pizza or a spicy curry, but she reminded herself of the repercussions and stuck to her pledge. Dining out with friends posed another challenge, as she browsed menus with caution and always made her dietary requirements clear. Olivia's confidence in her capacity to manage GERD through mindful eating rose with each passing day.

Her effort was not overlooked by people around her. Friends and relatives marveled at her fortitude and the beautiful meals she continued to prepare despite her dietary limitations. Olivia took delight in sharing her recipes and information, knowing that she was positively impacting not just her own life, but also the lives of those suffering with GERD.

WHAT IS GASTROESOPHAGEAL REFLUX DISEASE

GERD, or Gastroesophageal Reflux Disease, is a chronic illness in which stomach acid returns to the esophagus, causing irritation and inflammation. Here is a summary of GERD, including its causes, symptoms, treatment, risk factors, and preventive measures:

Causes of Gastroesophageal Reflux Disease

1. Weak Lower Esophageal Sphincter (LES): This muscular ring serves as a valve between the esophagus and stomach. When the stomach muscles weaken or relax abnormally, acid can reflux into the esophagus.

2. Hiatal Hernia: The upper section of the stomach protrudes through the diaphragm into the chest cavity, weakening the LES and contributing to GERD.

3. **Abnormalities in the Esophagus**: including hiatal hernia, esophageal spasms, and decreased clearance, can raise the risk of GERD.

4. **Gastroparesis**: Delayed stomach emptying increases the risk of acid reflux.

5. Diet and Lifestyle Factors: Certain meals (e.g., fatty or spicy, caffeine, alcohol), smoking, obesity, and reclining down after eating can all cause GERD symptoms.

Symptoms Gastroesophageal Reflux Disease

1. Heartburn is a burning sensation in the chest, typically after eating or at night.

2. Regurgitation refers to sour or bitter acid backing up into the throat or mouth.

3. Dysphagia refers to difficulty swallowing, or the sense of food stuck in the throat.

4. Chest Pain: GERD symptoms may mimic heart attack symptoms.

5. Chronic cough, particularly at night or in the morning.

6. Acid can cause hoarseness or a sore throat.

7. Dental Erosion: Acid reflux can wear away enamel over time.

Treatment of Gastroesophageal Reflux Disease

1. Lifestyle modifications include elevating the head of the bed, avoiding lying down after meals, decreasing weight (if overweight), quitting smoking, and avoiding trigger foods.

2. Adopt a GERD-friendly diet by minimizing trigger foods and increasing whole grains, lean meats, fruits, and vegetables.

3. Medications: Over-the-counter antacids, H2 receptor blockers (e.g., ranitidine), and proton pump inhibitors (e.g., omeprazole) can alleviate acid production and symptoms.

4. Surgery: In extreme situations or when drugs fail, fundoplication may be indicated to reinforce the LES and prevent reflux.

Risk Factors

1. Obesity: Excess weight exerts pressure on the abdomen, raising the risk of reflux.

2. Smoking weakens the LES and reduces saliva production, potentially worsening GERD symptoms.

3. Hiatal Hernia: People with hiatal hernias are more likely to experience GERD symptoms.

4. Pregnancy: Changes in hormones and abdominal pressure can raise the risk of GERD.

5. Certain medications: Some drugs, such as calcium channel blockers, antihistamines, and certain asthma treatments, can relax or irritate the esophagus.

Preventive Measures of Gastroesophageal Reflux Disease

1. Maintain a Healthy Weight: Losing extra weight helps relieve abdominal pressure and lower the risk of GERD symptoms.

2. Eating smaller, more frequent meals helps minimize overfilling and reduce reflux risk.

3. Identify and avoid trigger foods for GERD symptoms, such as spicy, fatty, or acidic foods.

4. Limit alcohol and caffeine, as these might relax the LES and cause acid reflux.

5. Quit smoking, as it weakens the LES and raises the risk of GERD symptoms.

6. Manage Stress: Meditation, yoga, and deep breathing exercises can help reduce stress and improve GERD symptoms.

7. Wait before lying down: Avoid going to bed just after eating. Allow at least 2-3 hours for digestion before laying down.

COMPLICATIONS OF UNTREATED GERD IN SENIORS

Untreated GERD (Gastroesophageal Reflux Disease) in seniors can result in a number of serious consequences, compromising their health and quality of life. Here are some possible complications:

1. Esophagitis: Chronic exposure to stomach acid can cause inflammation and irritation, resulting in esophagitis. This can cause pain, trouble swallowing, and even bleeding in severe situations.

2. Esophageal Stricture: Untreated GERD can induce inflammation and scarring, narrowing the esophagus over time, resulting in esophageal stricture. This can make swallowing difficult and increase the likelihood of food getting caught in the esophagus.

3. Barrett's Esophagus: Chronic GERD can alter the cells lining the lower esophagus, leading to the condition known as Barrett's Esophagus. Barrett's esophagus raises the chance of esophageal cancer, yet it remains quite low.

4. Esophageal Cancer: Untreated GERD may cause esophageal cancer, especially in those with Barrett's esophagus. Esophageal cancer is a dangerous, potentially fatal illness that demands immediate medical attention.

5. Respiratory Complications: GERD can worsen asthma, chronic cough, and recurring pneumonia. Stomach acid refluxing into the throat and airways can cause inflammation and irritation, exacerbating respiratory symptoms.

6. Dental Erosion: Prolonged contact to stomach acid can cause enamel erosion, increasing the risk of tooth damage, sensitivity, and loss.

7. Sleep Disturbances: GERD symptoms like heartburn and regurgitation might worsen at night, causing sleeplessness, frequent awakenings, and weariness throughout the day.

FOOD TO INCLUDE AND FOOD TO AVOID

Food to Include

1. Choose whole grains like oats, brown rice, quinoa, and whole wheat bread, which are high in fiber and reduce reflux.

2. Choose lean protein sources, such as poultry, fish, tofu, and lentils, as they are easier to digest and less prone to trigger reflux than fatty meats.

3. Non-Citrus Fruits: Bananas, apples, pears, and melons have lower acidity and are less prone to trigger GERD symptoms.

4. Consume non-acidic vegetables including leafy greens, broccoli, carrots, and sweet potatoes to boost vitamin, mineral, and antioxidant intake.

5. Low-Fat Dairy: Choose low-fat or non-fat dairy products like yogurt, milk, and cheese to deliver critical nutrients without aggravating reflux symptoms.

6. Use mild herbs and spices like ginger, turmeric, and parsley to flavor food without irritating the esophagus.

Food to Avoid

1. High-Fat Foods: Fried foods, fatty meats, and creamy sauces can relax the lower esophageal sphincter (LES), causing stomach acid to reflux into the esophagus.

2. Acidic foods, including citrus fruits and juices, tomatoes, and vinegar, can worsen GERD symptoms by irritating the esophagus and increasing acid production.

3. Spicy foods can cause acid reflux by irritating stomach and esophageal linings, resulting in discomfort and heartburn.

4. Chocolate and Caffeine: Chocolate can relax the LES, while caffeine can increase acid production, perhaps leading to GERD symptoms.

5. Carbonated beverages, such as soda and sparkling water, can cause bloating and gas, leading to reflux.

6. Mint and Peppermint: While mint has digestive advantages, it can relax the LES and increase GERD symptoms in some people.

7. Onions and garlic might trigger heartburn and reflux due to their high sulfur content.

Portion Control and Eating Habits

1. Eating smaller, more frequent meals can avoid overeating and minimize stomach pressure, lowering the risk of reflux.

2. Slow Eating: Chew food completely and slowly to avoid swallowing air, which can cause bloating and reflux.

3. Avoid Late-Night Eating: Eat as least 2-3 hours before bedtime to ensure good digestion and reduce reflux symptoms.

4. Remain upright for at least two hours after eating to reduce reflux. Avoid lying down or leaning over quickly after a meal.

5. Maintain a Healthy Weight: Excess weight can put strain on the abdomen, increasing the risk of reflux. Aim to maintain a healthy weight by engaging in regular exercise and eating a balanced diet.

CHAPTER 1

Breakfast Recipes

1. Berry and Banana Smoothie

Health Benefits

- Rich in antioxidants and vitamins from berries.

- High in potassium and fiber from bananas.

- It can be digested easily and gentle on the stomach.

Ingredients

- 1 ripe banana, sliced

- Mixed berries of 1/2 cup (such as strawberries, blueberries, and raspberries)

- Plain Greek yogurt of 1/2 cup (low-fat or non-fat)

- 1/2 cup unsweetened almond milk

- 1 tablespoon honey (optional)

- Ice cubes (optional)

Mode of Preparation

1. In a blender, combine the sliced banana, mixed berries, Greek yogurt, almond milk, and honey (if using).

2. Blend until smooth and creamy.

3. Ice cubes should be added if desired and blend again until well combined.

4. Pour into glasses and serve immediately.

Nutritional Information

- Calories: 150

- Protein: 7g

- Fat: 1g

- Carbohydrates: 30g

- Fiber: 5g

- Sugar: 18g

Serving Size: 1 smoothie

Preparation Time: 5 minutes

2. Oatmeal with Almond Butter and Sliced Apples

Health Benefits

- Oatmeal provides soluble fiber, which can help soothe the digestive tract.

- Almond butter is a good source of healthy fats and protein.

- Apples are low in acidity and high in fiber, aiding digestion.

Ingredients

- 1/2 cup old-fashioned oats

- Water or unsweetened almond milk of 1 cup

- 1 tablespoon almond butter

- 1/2 apple, thinly sliced

- Cinnamon (optional)

- Honey or maple syrup (optional)

Mode of Preparation

1. In a small saucepan, bring water or almond milk to a boil.

2. Stir in the oats and reduce heat to low. Cook for 5-7 minutes, stirring occasionally, until oats are soft and creamy.

3. Transfer the cooked oats to a bowl and top with almond butter, sliced apples, and a sprinkle of cinnamon.

4. Drizzle with honey or maple syrup if desired.

5. Serve warm.

Nutritional Information

- Calories: 280

- Protein: 9g

- Fat: 11g

- Carbohydrates: 40g

- Fiber: 7g

- Sugar: 12g

Serving Size: 1 bowl of oatmeal

Cooking Time: 10 minutes

Preparation Time: 5 minutes

3. Greek Yogurt Parfait with Granola and Berries

Health Benefits

- Greek yogurt is high in protein and calcium, aiding in digestion and bone health.

- Berries are rich in antioxidants and fiber, promoting digestive health.

- Granola adds crunch and additional fiber to the meal.

Ingredients

- Plain Greek yogurt of 1/2 cup (low-fat or non-fat)

- 1/4 cup granola (low-fat, low-sugar)

- 1/4 cup mixed berries (such as strawberries, blueberries, and raspberries)

- 1 tablespoon honey (optional)

Mode of Preparation

1. Layer Greek yogurt in a glass or bowl, granola, and mixed berries.

2. Layers should be repeated until all ingredients are used up.

3. Drizzle with honey if desired.

4. Serve immediately.

Nutritional Information

- Calories: 250

- Protein: 15g

- Fat: 5g

- Carbohydrates: 40g

- Fiber: 5g

- Sugar: 15g

Serving Size: 1 parfait

Preparation Time: 5 minutes

4. Scrambled Tofu with Spinach and Tomatoes

Health Benefits

- Tofu provides plant-based protein and is easy to digest.

- Spinach is rich in vitamins and minerals, including iron and magnesium.

- Tomatoes are low in acidity and high in lycopene, a powerful antioxidant.

Ingredients

- 1/2 block firm tofu, crumbled

- 1 cup fresh spinach leaves

- 1/2 cup cherry tomatoes, halved

- 1/4 teaspoon garlic powder

- Salt and pepper to taste

- Cooking spray or olive oil for cooking

Mode of Preparation

1. Non-stick skillet should be heated over medium heat and lightly coat with cooking spray or olive oil.

2. Add crumbled tofu to the skillet and cook for 2-3 minutes, stirring occasionally.

3. Add spinach leaves and cherry tomatoes to the skillet. Cook for an additional 2-3 minutes until spinach is wilted and tomatoes are softened.

4. It should be seasoned with garlic powder, salt, and pepper to taste.

5. It should be removed from heat and transfer to a plate.

6. Serve hot.

Nutritional Information

- Calories: 180

- Protein: 15g

- Fat: 10g

- Carbohydrates: 8g

- Fiber: 3g

- Sugar: 2g

Serving Size: 1 serving

Cooking Time: 10 minutes

Preparation Time: 5 minutes

5. Whole Wheat Toast with Avocado and Sliced Hard-Boiled Eggs

Health Benefits

- Whole wheat toast provides fiber and complex carbohydrates for sustained energy.

- Avocado is rich in healthy fats and potassium, supporting heart health.

- Hard-boiled eggs are a good source of protein and essential vitamins and minerals.

Ingredients

- 2 slices whole wheat bread, toasted

- 1/2 ripe avocado, mashed

- 2 hard-boiled eggs, sliced

- Salt and pepper to taste

- Red pepper flakes (optional)

Mode of Preparation

1. Spread mashed avocado evenly onto each slice of toasted whole wheat bread.

2. Arrange sliced hard-boiled eggs on top of the avocado.

3. Season with salt, pepper, and red pepper flakes if desired.

4. Serve immediately.

Nutritional Information

- Calories: 300

- Protein: 15g

- Fat: 15g

- Carbohydrates: 25g

- Fiber: 8g

- Sugar: 2g

Serving Size: 1 serving (2 slices of toast)

Cooking Time: 15 minutes (including boiling eggs)

Preparation Time: 5 minutes

6. Blueberry Almond Butter Overnight Oats

Health Benefits

- Oats provide soluble fiber, aiding digestion and promoting satiety.

- Blueberries are rich in antioxidants and vitamin C, supporting immune health.

- Almond butter adds healthy fats and protein, helping to stabilize blood sugar levels.

Ingredients

- 1/2 cup old-fashioned oats

- 1/2 cup unsweetened almond milk

- 1 tablespoon almond butter

- 1/4 cup fresh or frozen blueberries

- Honey of 1 tablespoon or maple syrup (optional)

- 1 tablespoon sliced almonds (optional)

Mode of Preparation

1. In a jar or container, combine oats, almond milk, almond butter, and blueberries.

2. Stir well to combine all ingredients.

3. Cover the jar or container and refrigerate overnight or for at least 4 hours.

4. Before serving, stir the mixture and add honey or maple syrup if desired.

5. Top with sliced almonds for added crunch.

6. Enjoy chilled.

Nutritional Information

- Calories: 300

- Protein: 9g

- Fat: 12g

- Carbohydrates: 40g

- Fiber: 6g

- Sugar: 9g

Serving Size: 1 serving

Preparation Time: 5 minutes

7. Spinach and Feta Egg Muffins

Health Benefits

- Eggs provide high-quality protein and essential nutrients like vitamin D and choline.

- Spinach is rich in vitamins A and K, as well as iron and calcium, supporting bone and immune health.

- Feta cheese adds flavor and calcium, contributing to bone health.

Ingredients

- 6 large eggs

- 1 cup fresh spinach, chopped

- 1/4 cup crumbled feta cheese

- Salt and pepper to taste

- Olive oil or cooking spray can be use for greasing muffin tin.

Mode of Preparation

1. Preheat the oven to 350°F (175°C) and lightly grease a muffin tin with cooking spray or olive oil.

2. In a mixing bowl, whisk together eggs, chopped spinach, crumbled feta cheese, salt, and pepper.

3. Pour the egg mixture evenly into the prepared muffin tin, filling each cup about 3/4 full.

4. Egg muffins should be baked in the preheated oven for 18-20 minutes, or they are set and lightly golden on top.

5. It should be removed from the oven and allow to cool slightly before serving.

6. Serve warm or at room temperature.

Nutritional Information

- Calories: 180
- Protein: 14g
- Fat: 12g
- Carbohydrates: 2g
- Fiber: 1g
- Sugar: 1g

Serving Size: 2 egg muffins

Cooking Time: 20 minutes

Preparation Time: 10 minutes

8. Quinoa Breakfast Bowl with Berries and Almonds

Health Benefits

- Quinoa is a complete protein and rich in fiber, supporting digestive health and providing sustained energy.

- Berries are high in antioxidants and vitamin C, promoting immune function and reducing inflammation.

- Almonds add healthy fats and protein, supporting heart health and satiety.

Ingredients

- 1/2 cup cooked quinoa

- 1/4 cup mixed berries (such as strawberries, blueberries, and raspberries)

- 1 tablespoon sliced almonds

- Honey of 1 tablespoon or maple syrup (optional)

- Cinnamon (optional)

Mode of Preparation

1. In a bowl, combine cooked quinoa, mixed berries, and sliced almonds.

2. It should be Drizzled with honey or maple syrup if desired.

3. Sprinkle with cinnamon for added flavor.

4. Stir gently to combine all ingredients.

5. Serve immediately.

Nutritional Information

- Calories: 250

- Protein: 8g

- Fat: 6g

- Carbohydrates: 40g

- Fiber: 6g

- Sugar: 15g

Serving Size: 1 bowl of quinoa breakfast

Cooking Time: 15 minutes (for cooking quinoa)

Preparation Time: 5 minutes

9. Banana Almond Pancakes

Health Benefits

- Bananas are rich in potassium and fiber, aiding digestion and supporting heart health.

- Almond flour provides protein and healthy fats, making these pancakes more filling and satisfying.

- These pancakes are gluten-free, making them suitable for individuals with gluten sensitivities.

Ingredients

- 1 ripe banana, mashed

- 2 eggs

- 1/4 cup almond flour

- 1/4 teaspoon baking powder

- 1/4 teaspoon cinnamon

- Cooking spray or coconut oil for cooking

Mode of Preparation

1. In a mixing bowl, whisk together mashed banana and eggs until well combined.

2. Add almond flour, baking powder, and cinnamon to the banana mixture. Stir until smooth.

3. Heat a non-stick skillet over medium heat and lightly coat with cooking spray or coconut oil.

4. Pour about 1/4 cup of the pancake batter onto the skillet for each pancake.

5. Cook for 2-3 minutes on each side, or until golden brown and cooked through.

6. Repeat with the remaining batter.

7. Serve the pancakes warm with sliced bananas, a drizzle of honey or maple syrup, and a sprinkle of cinnamon, if desired.

Nutritional Information

- Calories: 250

- Protein: 12g

- Fat: 12g

- Carbohydrates: 25g

- Fiber: 4g

- Sugar: 12g

Serving Size: 2 pancakes

Cooking Time: 10 minutes

Preparation Time: 10 minutes

10. Vegetable Frittata

Health Benefits

- Eggs provide high-quality protein and essential nutrients, supporting overall health and muscle function.

- Vegetables such as bell peppers, onions, and spinach are rich in vitamins, minerals, and antioxidants, promoting immune function and digestive health.

- This dish is low in carbohydrates and gluten-free, making it suitable for individuals with dietary restrictions.

Ingredients

- 6 large eggs

- Diced bell peppers of 1/2 cup (any color)

- 1/4 cup diced onion

- 1/2 cup chopped spinach

- Salt and pepper to taste

- Cooking spray or olive oil for cooking

Mode of Preparation

1. Preheat the oven to 350°F (175°C).

2. In a mixing bowl, whisk together eggs, diced bell peppers, diced onion, chopped spinach, salt, and pepper until well combined.

3. Heat a non-stick skillet over medium heat and lightly coat with cooking spray or olive oil.

4. Pour the egg mixture into the skillet and cook for 3-4 minutes, or until the edges begin to set.

5. Transfer the skillet to the preheated oven and bake for 10-12 minutes, or until the frittata is set and lightly golden on top.

6. Remove from the oven and allow to cool slightly before slicing.

7. Serve the frittata warm or at room temperature.

Nutritional Information

- Calories: 200

- Protein: 15g

- Fat: 10g

- Carbohydrates: 8g

- Fiber: 2g

- Sugar: 2g

Serving Size: 1/4 of the frittata

Cooking Time: 20 minutes

Preparation Time: 10 minutes

CHAPTER 2

Lunch Recipes

1. Grilled Chicken and Vegetable Salad
Health Benefits

- High in lean protein, which helps promote satiety and supports muscle health.

- Packed with fiber-rich vegetables that aid digestion and provide essential nutrients.

- Low in fat and acidity, making it gentle on the digestive system for GERD patients.

Ingredients

- Boneless and skinless chicken breasts (4) (about 6 ounces each)

- 2 cups mixed salad greens (e.g., spinach, arugula, romaine)

- 1 cup cherry tomatoes, halved

- 1 cucumber, sliced

- 1 bell pepper, thinly sliced

- 1/4 red onion, thinly sliced

- 2 tablespoons olive oil

- 1 tablespoon balsamic vinegar

- Salt and pepper to taste

Mode of Preparation

1. Grill or grill pan should be pre heated over medium-high heat.

2. Chicken breasts should be seasoned with salt and pepper.

3. Each side should be Grilled for 6-8 minutes until cooked through.

4. In a large bowl, combine salad greens, cherry tomatoes, cucumber, bell pepper, and red onion.

5. Whisk together olive oil and balsamic vinegar in a bowl to make the dressing.

6. Slice grilled chicken and add to the salad.

7. It should be Drizzled with dressing and toss to combine.

8. Serve immediately.

Nutritional Information

- Calories: 350

- Protein: 30g

- Carbohydrates: 12g

- Fat: 20g

- Fiber: 4g

Serving Size: 1 portion

Cooking Time: 15 minutes

Preparation Time: 10 minutes

2. Quinoa and Vegetable Stir-Fry

Health Benefits

- Quinoa is a complete protein source and provides essential amino acids for muscle repair and maintenance.

- Loaded with fiber from vegetables, aiding digestion and promoting gut health.

- Low in fat and acidity, suitable for GERD patients.

Ingredients

- 1 cup quinoa

- 2 cups water

- 1 tablespoon olive oil

- 2 cloves garlic, minced

- 1 bell pepper, chopped

- 1 cup broccoli florets

- 1 cup snow peas

- 1 carrot, sliced

- 2 tablespoons low-sodium soy sauce

- 1 teaspoon sesame oil

- Sesame seeds for garnish (optional)

Mode of Preparation

1. Rinse quinoa under cold water.

2. Combine quinoa and water in a saucepan.

3. It should be brought to a boil, then reduce heat to low, cover, and simmer for 15 minutes or until quinoa is cooked and water is absorbed.

4. Olive oil should be heated in a large skillet, over medium heat.

5. Minced garlic should be added and cook for 1 minute until fragrant.

6. Add bell pepper, broccoli, snow peas, and carrot to the skillet.

7. The vegetables should be Stir-fry for 5-7 minutes until they are tender-crisp.

8. It should be stirred in cooked quinoa, soy sauce, and sesame oil.

9. It should be cooked for an additional 2-3 minutes, stirring continuously.

10. Garnish with sesame seeds if desired before serving.

Nutritional Information

- Calories: 300

- Protein: 10g

- Carbohydrates: 45g

- Fat: 8g

- Fiber: 8g

Serving Size: 1 portion

Cooking Time: 20 minutes

Preparation Time: 15 minutes

3. Turkey and Avocado Wrap
Health Benefits

- Turkey is a lean protein source that aids in muscle maintenance and repair.

- Avocado provides healthy fats and fiber, promoting satiety and supporting heart health.

- This recipe is low in acidity and easy to digest, suitable for GERD patients.

Ingredients

- 4 whole grain tortillas

- 8 ounces sliced turkey breast

- 1 avocado, sliced

- 1 cup spinach leaves

- 1/2 cup sliced cucumber

- 1/4 cup Greek yogurt

- 1 tablespoon lemon juice

- Salt and pepper to taste

Mode of Preparation

1. In a small bowl, mix Greek yogurt and lemon juice to make the dressing. Season with salt and pepper.

2. Lay out tortillas and spread Greek yogurt dressing evenly on each.

3. Layer turkey slices, avocado slices, spinach leaves, and sliced cucumber on each tortilla.

4. Roll up tortillas tightly, tucking in the ends to secure
    the fillings.

5. Slice each wrap in half diagonally before serving.

Nutritional Information

- Calories: 300

- Protein: 25g

- Carbohydrates: 30g

- Fat: 10g

- Fiber: 8g

Serving Size: 1 wrap

Cooking Time: 10 minutes

Preparation Time: 10 minutes

4. Lentil Soup with Spinach

Health Benefits

- Lentils are rich in protein and fiber, promoting satiety and aiding digestion.

- Spinach provides essential vitamins and minerals, including iron and folate, supporting overall health.

- This soup is low in fat and acidity, making it gentle on the stomach for GERD patients.

Ingredients

- 1 cup dried green lentils

- 4 cups low-sodium vegetable broth

- 1 onion, diced

- 2 carrots, diced

- 2 celery stalks, diced

- 2 cloves garlic, minced

- 1 teaspoon ground cumin

- 1/2 teaspoon paprika

- Salt and pepper to taste

- 2 cups fresh spinach leaves

Mode of Preparation

1. The lentils should be rinsed under cold water and drain.

2. In a large pot, heat vegetable broth over medium heat. Add diced onion, carrots, celery, and minced garlic.

3. It should be cooked for 5-7 minutes until vegetables are softened.

4. Stir in lentils, ground cumin, paprika, salt, and pepper.

5. It should be brought to a boil, then reduce heat to low, cover, and simmer for 20-25 minutes until lentils are tender.

6. Add fresh spinach leaves to the soup and cook for an additional 2-3 minutes until wilted.

7. Adjust seasoning if needed before serving.

Nutritional Information

- Calories: 200

- Protein: 12g

- Carbohydrates: 35g

- Fat: 1g

- Fiber: 12g

Serving Size: 1 cup

Cooking Time: 30 minutes

Preparation Time: 15 minutes

5. Baked Salmon with Steamed Vegetables

Health Benefits

- Salmon contains omega-3 fatty acids, which promote heart health and prevent inflammation.

- Steamed vegetables provide vitamins, minerals, and fiber, supporting overall health and digestion.

- This dish is low in fat and acidity, making it suitable for GERD patients.

Ingredients

- Salmon fillets of 4

- 1 lemon, thinly sliced

- Mixed vegetables of 2 cups (e.g., broccoli, cauliflower, carrots)

- 2 teaspoons olive oil

- Salt and pepper to taste

- Fresh dill for garnish (optional)

Mode of Preparation

1. Preheat oven to 375°F (190°C).

2. Baking sheet should be lined with parchment paper.

3. Salmon fillets should be placed on the prepared baking sheet. Season with salt and pepper to taste.

4. Lemon slices should be arranged on top of the salmon.

5. Bake salmon in the preheated oven for 12-15 minutes until cooked through and flaky.

6. Meanwhile, steam mixed vegetables until tender-crisp, about 5-7 minutes.

7. Drizzle steamed vegetables with olive oil and season with salt and pepper.

8. Serve baked salmon alongside steamed vegetables. Garnish with fresh dill if desired.

Nutritional Information

- Calories: 350

- Protein: 30g

- Carbohydrates: 10g

- Fat: 20g

- Fiber: 5g

Serving Size: 1 salmon fillet with vegetables

Cooking Time: 20 minutes

Preparation Time: 10 minutes

6. Turkey and Quinoa Stuffed Bell Peppers

Health Benefits

- Lean turkey provides protein for muscle health without excess fat.

- Quinoa offers fiber and essential nutrients while being gentle on the digestive system.

- Bell peppers are low in acidity and provide vitamins and antioxidants.

Ingredients

- 4 large bell peppers (any color)

- 1 cup cooked quinoa

- 8 ounces ground turkey

- 1 small onion, diced

- 2 cloves garlic, minced

- 1 teaspoon olive oil

- 1 teaspoon Italian seasoning

- Salt and pepper to taste

- 1/2 cup low-sodium tomato sauce

- 1/2 cup shredded mozzarella cheese

Mode of Preparation

1. Preheat oven to 375°F (190°C).

2. The top of bell peppers should be sliced off and remove seeds and membranes.

3. Skillet should be used for heating Olive over medium heat.

4. Add diced onion and minced garlic, sauté until softened.

5. Ground turkey should be added to the skillet, and break it up with a spoon, and cook until browned.

6. It should be seasoned with Italian seasoning, salt, and pepper.

7. Stir in cooked quinoa and tomato sauce, mixing until well combined.

8. Stuff each bell pepper with the turkey-quinoa mixture and place them upright in a baking dish.

9. Baking dish should be covered with foil and bake for 25 minutes.

10. The Foil should be removed, sprinkle shredded mozzarella cheese over the stuffed peppers, and bake for an additional 10 minutes until cheese is melted and bubbly.

11. Serve hot.

Nutritional Information

- Calories: 300

- Protein: 25g

- Carbohydrates: 25g

- Fat: 12g

- Fiber: 5g

Serving Size: 1 stuffed bell pepper

Cooking Time: 45 minutes

Preparation Time: 20 minutes

7. Veggie and Hummus Wrap
Health Benefits

- Hummus provides plant-based protein and healthy fats, aiding satiety and promoting heart health.

- Colorful vegetables offer vitamins, minerals, and fiber while being low in acidity.

- This wrap is light and easy to digest, suitable for GERD patients.

Ingredients

- 4 whole grain wraps or tortillas

- 1 cup hummus

- 2 cups mixed salad greens

- 1 cucumber, thinly sliced

- 1 bell pepper, thinly sliced

- 1 carrot, grated

- 1/4 cup sliced black olives (optional)

- Salt and pepper to taste

Mode of Preparation

1. Lay out wraps or tortillas on a clean surface.

2. Generous amount of hummus should be evenly spread on each wrap.

3. Layer mixed salad greens, cucumber slices, bell pepper slices, grated carrot, and sliced black olives (if using) on each wrap.

4. Salt and pepper should be added to taste.

5. Roll up wraps tightly, tucking in the ends to secure the fillings.

6. Slice each wrap in half diagonally before serving.

Nutritional Information

- Calories: 250

- Protein: 10g

- Carbohydrates: 35g

- Fat: 8g

- Fiber: 8g

Serving Size: 1 wrap

Cooking Time: 10 minutes

Preparation Time: 10 minutes

8. Tuna Salad Lettuce Wraps

Health Benefits

- Tuna is a lean protein source rich in omega-3 fatty acids, supporting heart health and reducing inflammation.

- Lettuce leaves provide a low-acid alternative to bread while offering vitamins and minerals.

- This recipe is light, refreshing, and easy to digest, making it suitable for GERD patients.

Ingredients

- Tuna of 2 cans (5 ounces each), drained

- 1/4 cup Greek yogurt

- 1 tablespoon lemon juice

- 1/4 cup diced celery

- 1/4 cup diced red onion

- 1 tablespoon chopped fresh dill

- Salt and pepper to taste

- 8 large lettuce leaves (e.g., romaine or butter lettuce)

Mode of Preparation

1. In a bowl, combine drained tuna, Greek yogurt, lemon juice, diced celery, diced red onion, and chopped fresh dill. Mix until well combined.

2. Season tuna salad with salt and pepper to taste.

3. Place a spoonful of tuna salad onto each lettuce leaf.

4. Roll up lettuce leaves, enclosing the filling, to create wraps.

5. Serve chilled.

Nutritional Information

- Calories: 200

- Protein: 20g

- Carbohydrates: 5g

- Fat: 8g

- Fiber: 2g

Serving Size: 2 lettuce wraps

Cooking Time: 10 minutes

Preparation Time: 10 minutes

9. Veggie and Turkey Lettuce Wraps
Health Benefits

- Lean turkey provides protein for muscle health without excess fat.

- Colorful vegetables offer vitamins, minerals, and fiber while being low in acidity.

- Lettuce leaves provide a low-acid alternative to bread, making this recipe gentle on the digestive system for GERD patients.

Ingredients

- 1 pound lean ground turkey

- 1 tablespoon olive oil

- 1 onion, diced

- 2 cloves garlic, minced

- 1 bell pepper, diced

- 1 zucchini, diced

- 1 carrot, grated

- 1 teaspoon ground cumin

- 1 teaspoon paprika

- Salt and pepper to taste

- 8 large lettuce leaves (e.g., romaine or butter lettuce)

Mode of Preparation

1. Olive oil should be heated in a large skillet over medium heat. Add diced onion and minced garlic, sauté until softened.

2. Add ground turkey to the skillet, breaking it up with a spoon, and cook until browned.

3. Stir in diced bell pepper, diced zucchini, grated carrot, ground cumin, paprika, salt, and pepper.

4. It should be cooked for 5-7 minutes until vegetables are tender.

5. Turkey and vegetable mixture should be spoon onto each lettuce leaf.

6. Roll up lettuce leaves, enclosing the filling, to create wraps.

7. Serve warm.

Nutritional Information

- Calories: 300

- Protein: 25g

- Carbohydrates: 10g

- Fat: 15g

- Fiber: 4g

Serving Size: 2 lettuce wraps

Cooking Time: 20 minutes

Preparation Time: 15 minutes

10. Baked Cod with Lemon and Herbs

Health Benefits

- Cod is a lean source of protein that's easy to digest and gentle on the stomach.

- Lemon and herbs provide flavor without adding excess fat or acidity, making this dish suitable for GERD patients.

Ingredients

- Cod fillets (4)

- 2 tablespoons olive oil

- 2 tablespoons fresh lemon juice

- 2 cloves garlic, minced

- 1 tablespoon chopped fresh parsley

- 1 tablespoon chopped fresh dill

- Salt and pepper to taste

- Lemon slices for garnish (optional)

Mode of Preparation

1. Preheat oven to 375°F (190°C). Line a baking dish with parchment paper.

2. Cod fillets should be placed in the prepared baking dish.

3. It should be Drizzled with olive oil and lemon juice.

4. Sprinkle minced garlic, chopped fresh parsley, chopped fresh dill, salt, and pepper evenly over the cod fillets.

5. Bake in the preheated oven for 15-20 minutes until fish is opaque and flakes easily with a fork.

6. Garnish with lemon slices before serving.

Nutritional Information

- Calories: 200

- Protein: 30g

- Carbohydrates: 1g

- Fat: 8g

- Fiber: 0g

Serving Size: 1 cod fillet

Cooking Time: 20 minutes

Preparation Time: 10 minutes

CHAPTER 3

Dinner Recipes

1: Baked Salmon with Lemon-Dill Sauce

Health Benefits

- Salmon is rich in omega-3 fatty acids, which have anti-inflammatory properties that may help reduce GERD symptoms.

- Lemon provides vitamin C and adds flavor without acidity.

- Dill is a natural digestive aid and adds a refreshing touch to the dish.

Ingredients

- Salmon fillets (4) (6 ounces each).

- 2 tablespoons olive oil

- Salt and pepper to taste

- 1 lemon, sliced

- 2 tablespoons chopped fresh dill

Mode of Preparation

1. Preheat the oven to 375°F (190°C).

2. Baking sheet should be lined with parchment paper.

3. Salmon fillets should be placed on the prepared baking sheet.

4. It should be Drizzled with olive oil and season with salt and pepper.

5. Top each fillet with lemon slices and sprinkle with chopped dill.

6. It should be baked in the preheated oven for 12-15 minutes, or until the salmon is cooked through and flakes easily with a fork.

7. Serve hot with additional lemon slices and dill, if desired.

Nutritional Information

- Calories: 320 kcal

- Protein: 34g

- Fat: 18g

- Carbohydrates: 2g

- Fiber: 1g

- Sodium: 120mg

Serving Size: 1 salmon fillet

Cooking Time: 12-15 minutes

Preparation Time: 10 minutes

2: Quinoa Salad with Grilled Chicken

Health Benefits

- Quinoa is a gluten-free whole grain rich in fiber, which aids digestion and promotes satiety.

- Grilled chicken breast provides lean protein without added fat, making it gentle on the stomach.

- Vegetables like cucumber and bell peppers add vitamins and minerals while being low in acidity.

Ingredients

- 1 cup quinoa

- Water of 2 Cups or low-sodium chicken broth

- 2 boneless, skinless chicken breasts

- 1 tablespoon olive oil

- Salt and pepper to taste

- 1 cucumber, diced

- 1 bell pepper (any color), diced

- 1/4 cup chopped fresh parsley

- Juice of 1 lemon

Mode of Preparation

1. Rinse quinoa under cold water.

2. Water of chicken broth should be brought to a boil in a medium saucepan.

3. Add quinoa, reduce heat to low, cover, and simmer for 15 minutes or until water is absorbed.

4. It should be brought down from heat and let stand for 5 minutes. Fluff with a fork.

5. Preheat grill or grill pan over medium-high heat.

6. Chicken breasts should be brushed with olive oil and season with salt and pepper.

7. It should be grilled for 6-8 minutes per side, or until cooked through.

8. Allow it to rest for 5 minutes before slicing.

9. In a large bowl, combine cooked quinoa, diced cucumber, diced bell pepper, chopped parsley, and lemon juice. Toss to combine.

10. Serve quinoa salad topped with sliced grilled chicken breast.

Nutritional Information

- Calories: 380 kcal

- Protein: 30g

- Fat: 10g

- Carbohydrates: 40g

- Fiber: 5g

- Sodium: 100mg

Serving Size: 1/4 of the recipe

Cooking Time: 25 minutes (including quinoa cooking time)

Preparation Time: 15 minutes

3: Turkey Meatballs with Zucchini Noodles

Health Benefits

- Lean ground turkey provides protein without excess fat, making it easy to digest.

- Zucchini noodles are a low-carb alternative to traditional pasta, reducing the risk of reflux.

- Garlic and herbs add flavor without added acidity.

Ingredients

- 1 lb lean ground turkey

- 1/4 cup breadcrumbs (gluten-free if desired)

- 1 egg

- 2 cloves garlic, minced

- 2 tablespoons chopped fresh parsley

- 1 teaspoon dried oregano

- Salt and pepper to taste

- 4 medium zucchini, spiralized into noodles

- 2 cups marinara sauce (low-acid variety)

Mode of Preparation

1. Preheat the oven to 400°F (200°C).

2. Baking sheet should be lined with parchment paper.

3. In a large bowl, combine ground turkey, breadcrumbs, egg, minced garlic, chopped parsley, dried oregano, salt, and pepper. Mix until well combined.

4. The mixture should be shaped into meatballs (about 1 inch in diameter) and place them on the prepared baking sheet.

5. It should be baked in the preheated oven for 20-25 minutes, or until the meatballs are cooked through and browned.

6. While the meatballs are baking, spiralize the zucchini into noodles using a spiralizer.

7. In a large skillet, heat marinara sauce over medium heat. Add zucchini noodles and cook for 3-4 minutes, or until tender.

8. Serve turkey meatballs over zucchini noodles topped with additional marinara sauce, if desired.

Nutritional Information

- Calories: 280 kcal

- Protein: 25g

- Fat: 10g

- Carbohydrates: 20g

- Fiber: 5g

- Sodium: 480mg

Serving Size: 4 meatballs with zucchini noodles

Cooking Time: 25 minutes

Preparation Time: 15 minutes

4: Vegetable Stir-Fry with Tofu

Health Benefits

- Tofu provides plant-based protein without added fat, making it a gentle option for GERD patients.

- Colorful vegetables like bell peppers, broccoli, and carrots provide vitamins, minerals, and antioxidants while being low in acidity.

- Stir-frying preserves the nutrients in vegetables while minimizing added fats.

Ingredients

- Firm tofu of 1 block, pressed and cubed

- 2 tablespoons low-sodium soy sauce (or tamari for gluten-free)

- 1 tablespoon sesame oil

- 2 cloves garlic, minced

- 1 tablespoon grated ginger

- 1 bell pepper (any color), sliced

- 1 cup broccoli florets

- 1 carrot, julienned

- 2 green onions, sliced

- Cooked brown rice or quinoa for serving

Mode of Preparation

1. In a small bowl, combine cubed tofu, soy sauce, sesame oil, minced garlic, and grated ginger. Let marinate for 15-20 minutes.

2. Large skillet or wok should be heated over medium-high heat. Add marinated tofu and cook for 5-6 minutes, or until golden brown.

3. Tofu should be remove from the skillet and set aside.

4. In the same skillet, add sliced bell pepper, broccoli florets, and julienned carrot.

5. The Vegetables should be Stir-fry or until they are tender-crisp.

6. Return cooked tofu to the skillet and add sliced green onions.

7. It should be cooked for an additional 1-2 minutes, stirring to combine.

- 1 bay leaf

- 2 cups fresh spinach leaves

- Salt and pepper to taste

Mode of Preparation

1. In a large pot, combine dried lentils, vegetable broth, diced onion, diced carrots, diced celery, minced garlic, dried thyme, dried rosemary, and bay leaf.

2. It should be brought to a boil over medium-high heat.

3. Reduce heat to low, cover, and simmer for 25-30 minutes, or until lentils and vegetables are tender.

4. Stir in fresh spinach leaves and cook for an additional 2-3 minutes, or until wilted.

5. It should be seasoned with salt and pepper to taste.

6. Remove bay leaf before serving.

Nutritional Information

- Calories: 250 kcal

- Protein: 15g

- Fat: 1g

- Carbohydrates: 45g

- Fiber: 15g

- Sodium: 500mg

Serving Size: 1 1/2 cups

Cooking Time: 35 minutes

Preparation Time: 10 minutes

6: Grilled Chicken and Vegetable Skewers

Health Benefits

- Grilled chicken provides lean protein without excess fat, making it easy to digest.

- Colorful vegetables like bell peppers, zucchini, and cherry tomatoes add vitamins, minerals, and fiber to the dish.

- Grilling preserves the nutrients in vegetables while minimizing added fats.

Ingredients

- Chicken breasts that is boneless and skinless (2), cut into cubes

- Cut into chunks 1 red bell pepper.

- 1 yellow bell pepper should be cut into chunks

- 1 zucchini, sliced into rounds

- 1 cup cherry tomatoes

- 2 tablespoons olive oil

- 2 cloves garlic, minced

- Chopped fresh herbs of 1 tablespoon (such as rosemary or thyme)

- Salt and pepper to taste

- Wooden skewers should be soaked in water for 30 minutes.

Mode of Preparation

1. In a bowl, combine cubed chicken, bell peppers, zucchini, cherry tomatoes, olive oil, minced garlic, chopped herbs, salt, and pepper. Toss until evenly coated.

2. Marinated chicken and vegetables should be thread onto the soaked wooden skewers, alternating between ingredients.

3. Preheat grill or grill pan over medium-high heat.

4. Grill the skewers for 8-10 minutes, turning occasionally, until the chicken is cooked through and the vegetables are tender.

5. Serve hot with a side of cooked quinoa or brown rice, if desired.

Nutritional Information

- Calories: 280 kcal

- Protein: 25g

- Fat: 12g

- Carbohydrates: 15g

- Fiber: 4g

- Sodium: 200mg

Serving Size: 2 skewers

Cooking Time: 10 minutes

Preparation Time: 20 minutes

7: Turkey and Vegetable Stir-Fry with Brown Rice

Health Benefits

- Lean ground turkey provides protein without excess fat, making it gentle on the stomach.

- Colorful vegetables like broccoli, bell peppers, and snap peas add vitamins, minerals, and fiber to the dish.

- Stir-frying preserves the nutrients in vegetables while minimizing added fats.

Ingredients

- 1 lb lean ground turkey

- 2 cups mixed vegetables (such as broccoli florets, bell peppers, snap peas)

- 2 cloves garlic, minced

- 1 tablespoon grated ginger

- 2 tablespoons low-sodium soy sauce (or tamari for gluten-free)

- 1 tablespoon sesame oil

- Cooked brown rice for serving

Mode of Preparation

1. Large skillet or wok should be heated over medium-high heat. Add ground turkey and cook until browned, breaking it up with a spoon.

2. Add minced garlic and grated ginger to the skillet and cook for 1-2 minutes, until fragrant.

3. Add mixed vegetables to the skillet and stir-fry for 3-4 minutes, or until tender-crisp.

4. Stir in low-sodium soy sauce and sesame oil, tossing to coat the turkey and vegetables evenly.

5. Serve hot over cooked brown rice.

Nutritional Information

- Calories: 320 kcal

- Protein: 25g

- Fat: 15g

- Carbohydrates: 20g

- Fiber: 4g

- Sodium: 450mg

Serving Size: 1/4 of the recipe

Cooking Time: 15 minutes

Preparation Time: 15 minutes

8: Veggie and Lentil Stuffed Bell Peppers

Health Benefits

- Lentils provide plant-based protein and fiber, promoting satiety and aiding digestion.

- Colorful bell peppers are rich in vitamins and minerals while being low in acidity.

- Baking preserves the nutrients in vegetables without adding excess fats.

Ingredients

- Big bell peppers (4), halved and seeds removed

- Dried green or brown lentils of 1 cup, rinsed and drained

- 2 cups vegetable broth

- 1 onion, diced

- 2 cloves garlic, minced

- 1 carrot, diced

- 1 stalk celery, diced

- 1 cup diced tomatoes (fresh or canned)

- 1 teaspoon dried oregano

- 1 teaspoon dried basil

- Salt and pepper to taste

- 1/2 cup shredded mozzarella cheese (optional)

Mode of Preparation

1. Preheat the oven to 375°F (190°C). Arrange halved bell peppers in a baking dish.

2. In a saucepan, combine dried lentils and vegetable broth. Bring to a boil, then reduce heat to low and simmer for 20-25 minutes, or until lentils are tender.

3. Olive oil should be heated in a large skillet over medium heat.

4. Diced onion, minced garlic, diced carrot, and diced celery should be added. Cook for 5-6 minutes, or until vegetables are softened.

5. Add cooked lentils, diced tomatoes, dried oregano, dried basil, salt, and pepper to the skillet.

6. Mix thoroughly so that it can combine and cook for an additional 2-3 minutes.

7. Spoon the lentil mixture into the halved bell peppers, dividing evenly. Top with shredded mozzarella cheese, if desired.

8. Cover the baking dish with foil and bake in the preheated oven for 25-30 minutes, or until the bell peppers are tender and the filling is heated through.

9. Serve hot as a main dish or with a side salad.

Nutritional Information

- Calories: 280 kcal

- Protein: 15g

- Fat: 5g

- Carbohydrates: 40g

- Fiber: 10g

- Sodium: 400mg

Serving Size: 1 stuffed bell pepper (2 halves)

Cooking Time: 30 minutes

Preparation Time: 20 minutes

9: Ginger-Garlic Shrimp Stir-Fry
Health Benefits

- Shrimp is a lean protein source and easily digestible, making it suitable for individuals with GERD.

- Ginger and garlic aids digestion because they contain anti-inflammatory properties.

- Stir-frying vegetables preserves their nutrients while minimizing added fats.

Ingredients

- Medium shrimp of 1 lb, peeled and deveined

- 2 tablespoons low-sodium soy sauce (or tamari for gluten-free)

- 1 tablespoon rice vinegar

- 1 tablespoon grated ginger

- 2 cloves garlic, minced

- 1 tablespoon sesame oil

- Mixed vegetables of 2 cups (such as bell peppers, snap peas, carrots)

- Cooked brown rice for serving

Mode of Preparation

1. In a bowl, combine shrimp, low-sodium soy sauce, rice vinegar, grated ginger, and minced garlic. Let marinate for 15-20 minutes.

2. Sesame oil should be heated in a large skillet or wok over medium-high heat. Add marinated shrimp and stir-fry for 2-3 minutes, or until pink and cooked through.

3. Shrimp should be removed from the skillet and set aside.

4. In the same skillet, add mixed vegetables and stir-fry for 3-4 minutes, or until tender-crisp.

5. Return cooked shrimp to the skillet and toss with the vegetables until heated through.

6. Serve hot over cooked brown rice.

Nutritional Information

- Calories: 250 kcal

- Protein: 25g

- Fat: 5g

- Carbohydrates: 25g

- Fiber: 5g

- Sodium: 400mg

Serving Size: 1/4 of the recipe

Cooking Time: 15 minutes

Preparation Time: 20 minutes

10: Roasted Vegetable and Chicken Sausage Quinoa Bowl

Health Benefits

- Chicken sausage provides lean protein with fewer saturated fats compared to pork sausage.

- Roasting vegetables caramelizes their natural sugars and enhances their flavors without adding excess fats.

- Quinoa is a gluten-free whole grain rich in fiber, promoting digestive health.

Ingredients

- 4 chicken sausage links (such as apple or spinach flavor), sliced

- 2 cups mixed vegetables (such as bell peppers, broccoli, cherry tomatoes)

- 1 tablespoon olive oil

- Salt and pepper to taste

- 1 cup quinoa

- 2 cups low-sodium chicken broth

- 1/4 cup chopped fresh parsley (optional)

- Lemon wedges for serving

Mode of Preparation

1. Preheat the oven to 400°F (200°C). Line a baking sheet with parchment paper.

2. In a bowl, toss sliced chicken sausage and mixed vegetables with olive oil, salt, and pepper until evenly coated.

3. It should be Spread onto the already prepared baking sheet in a single layer.

4. Roast in the preheated oven for 20-25 minutes, or until sausage is browned and vegetables are tender.

5. While the sausage and vegetables are roasting, rinse quinoa under cold water. In a saucepan, combine quinoa and low-sodium chicken broth.

6. It should be brought to a boil, then reduce heat to low, cover, and simmer for 15 minutes, or until quinoa is cooked and liquid is absorbed.

7. Fluff quinoa with a fork and divide among serving bowls. Top with roasted chicken sausage and

vegetables. Sprinkle with chopped parsley, if desired, and serve with lemon wedges for squeezing.

Nutritional Information

- Calories: 350 kcal

- Protein: 20g

- Fat: 10g

- Carbohydrates: 45g

- Fiber: 6g

- Sodium: 500mg

Serving Size: 1/4 of the recipe

Cooking Time: 25 minutes

Preparation Time: 15 minutes

CHAPTER 4

Snacks and Appetizer

1: Greek Yogurt Parfait with Berries

Health Benefits

- Greek yogurt is a rich source of protein, which can help promote satiety and stabilize blood sugar levels.

- Berries are high in antioxidants, vitamins, and fiber, which support digestive health and reduce inflammation.

Ingredients

- 1 cup Greek yogurt (plain, low-fat or non-fat)

- Mixed berries of 1/2 cup (such as strawberries, blueberries, raspberries)

- 2 tablespoons honey or maple syrup (optional)

- 1/4 cup granola (low-fat, low-sugar)

Mode of Preparation

1. In a small bowl or glass, layer Greek yogurt followed by a spoonful of mixed berries.

2. It should be Drizzled with honey or maple syrup if desired.

3. Repeat the layers until the bowl or glass is filled.

4. Top with granola for added texture and crunch.

Nutritional Information

- Calories: 200

- Protein: 10g

- Carbohydrates: 30g

- Fat: 5g

- Fiber: 4g

Serving Size: 1 parfait

Preparation Time: 5 minutes

2: Apple Slices with Almond Butter

Health Benefits

- Apples are a good source of fiber, which aids digestion and helps prevent constipation.

- Almond butter provides healthy fats and protein, promoting satiety and stabilizing blood sugar levels.

Ingredients

- 1 medium apple, sliced

- 2 tablespoons almond butter (unsweetened)

Mode of Preparation

1. Wash and slice the apple into thin wedges.

2. Almond butter should be spread on each apple slice.

Nutritional Information

- Calories: 180

- Protein: 4g

- Carbohydrates: 20g

- Fat: 10g

- Fiber: 6g

Serving Size: 1 medium apple with almond butter

Preparation Time: 5 minutes

3: Rice Cakes with Cottage Cheese and Tomato

Health Benefits

- Rice cakes provide a light and crunchy base that is easy to digest.

- Cottage cheese is a low-fat source of protein and calcium, supporting muscle health and bone strength.

- Tomatoes are low in acidity and high in antioxidants, supporting digestive health and reducing inflammation.

Ingredients

- 2 rice cakes (unsalted, plain)

- 1/2 cup low-fat cottage cheese

- 1 small tomato, sliced

- Fresh basil leaves, for garnish (optional)

Mode of Preparation

1. Spread cottage cheese evenly on each rice cake.

2. Top with sliced tomatoes.

3. It should be garnished with fresh basil leaves if desired.

Nutritional Information

- Calories: 150

- Protein: 10g

- Carbohydrates: 20g

- Fat: 2g

- Fiber: 2g

Serving Size: 2 rice cakes with cottage cheese and tomato

Preparation Time: 5 minutes

4: Baked Sweet Potato Chips

Health Benefits

- Sweet potatoes are rich in fiber and vitamins, supporting digestive health and immune function.

- Baking instead of frying reduces the fat content, making this snack lighter and easier to digest.

Ingredients

- 2 medium sweet potatoes, thinly sliced

- 1 tablespoon olive oil

- 1/2 teaspoon sea salt

- 1/2 teaspoon paprika (optional)

Mode of Preparation

1. Oven should be preheated to 375°F (190°C) and line a baking sheet with parchment paper.

2. In a large bowl, toss sweet potato slices with olive oil, sea salt, and paprika (if using).

3. Arrange the sweet potato slices in a single layer on the prepared baking sheet.

4. Bake for 15-20 minutes or until the edges are crispy and golden brown.

5. Allow to cool before serving.

Nutritional Information

- Calories: 120

- Protein: 2g

- Carbohydrates: 20g

- Fat: 4g

- Fiber: 4g

Serving Size: 1 cup of sweet potato chips

Cooking Time: 15-20 minutes

Preparation Time: 10 minutes

5: Cucumber and Hummus Rolls

Health Benefits

- Cucumbers are hydrating and low in acidity, making them gentle on the stomach.

- Hummus provides plant-based protein and fiber, promoting satiety and digestive health.

Ingredients

- 1 large cucumber

- 1/4 cup hummus (store-bought or homemade)

Mode of Preparation

1. Wash the cucumber and slice it lengthwise into thin strips using a vegetable peeler or mandoline slicer.

2. Thin layer of hummus should be spread onto each cucumber strip.

3. Roll up the cucumber strips and secure with toothpicks if necessary.

Nutritional Information

- Calories: 80

- Protein: 3g

- Carbohydrates: 10g

- Fat: 4g

- Fiber: 3g

Serving Size: 4 cucumber rolls

Preparation Time: 10 minutes

6: Vegetable Crudité with Yogurt Dip
Health Benefits

- Assorted vegetables provide vitamins, minerals, and fiber, supporting digestive health and overall well-being.

- Yogurt dip offers probiotics, which promote a healthy gut microbiome and aid in digestion.

Ingredients

- Assorted raw vegetables (carrots, celery, bell peppers, cucumber, cherry tomatoes, broccoli florets)

- 1 cup plain Greek yogurt

- 1 tablespoon lemon juice

- 1 teaspoon minced garlic

- Salt and pepper to taste

- Herbs that is fresh can be used for garnish but its optional.

Mode of Preparation

1. Wash and prepare the vegetables by cutting them into sticks or bite-sized pieces.

2. In a small bowl, whisk together the Greek yogurt, lemon juice, minced garlic, salt, and pepper to make the dip.

3. Arrange the vegetable crudité on a serving platter alongside the yogurt dip.

4. Garnish with fresh herbs if desired.

Nutritional Information

- Calories: 60

- Protein: 5g

- Carbohydrates: 8g

- Fat: 1g

- Fiber: 3g

Serving Size: 1 cup of vegetable crudité with dip

Preparation Time: 15 minutes

7: Baked Zucchini Fries

Health Benefits

- Zucchini is low in acidity and high in water content, making it gentle on the stomach.

- Baking instead of frying reduces the fat content, making this appetizer lighter and easier to digest.

Ingredients

- Zucchinis of medium size (2), cut into fry-shaped sticks

- 1/2 cup whole wheat breadcrumbs

- 1/4 cup grated Parmesan cheese

- 1 teaspoon garlic powder

- 1/2 teaspoon dried oregano

- 1/2 teaspoon paprika

- Salt and pepper to taste

- 1 egg, beaten

- Cooking spray

Mode of Preparation

1. Oven should be pre heated to 425°F (220°C) and baking sheet should be line with parchment paper

2. In a shallow dish, combine the breadcrumbs, Parmesan cheese, garlic powder, oregano, paprika, salt, and pepper.

3. Each zucchini stick should be dipped into the beaten egg, then coat with the breadcrumb mixture, pressing gently to adhere.

4. Place the coated zucchini sticks on the prepared baking sheet and spray lightly with cooking spray.

5. Bake for 20-25 minutes or until golden brown and crispy, flipping halfway through.

Nutritional Information

- Calories: 120

- Protein: 6g

- Carbohydrates: 15g

- Fat: 4g

- Fiber: 3g

Serving Size: 1 cup of zucchini fries

Cooking Time: 20-25 minutes

Preparation Time: 15 minutes

8: Melon and Prosciutto Skewers

Health Benefits

- Melons are hydrating and low in acidity, making them gentle on the stomach.

- Prosciutto provides protein and flavor without adding excess fat, making it a lighter option for appetizers.

Ingredients

- 1/2 small cantaloupe, cut into cubes

- 1/2 small honeydew melon, cut into cubes

- 4 slices prosciutto, cut into strips

- 8 wooden skewers

Mode of Preparation

1. Thread alternating pieces of cantaloupe, honeydew melon, and prosciutto onto each skewer.

2. Arrange the skewers on a serving platter and serve chilled.

Nutritional Information

- Calories: 80

- Protein: 5g

- Carbohydrates: 10g

- Fat: 3g

- Fiber: 1g

Serving Size: 2 skewers

Preparation Time: 10 minutes

9: Caprese Salad Skewers

Health Benefits

- Tomatoes are low in acidity and high in antioxidants, supporting digestive health.

- Mozzarella cheese provides protein and calcium, promoting bone health and muscle function.

- Basil offers anti-inflammatory properties and adds flavor without adding extra calories.

Ingredients

- 1 cup cherry tomatoes

- 1 cup mini fresh mozzarella balls (bocconcini)

- Fresh basil leaves

- Balsamic glaze (optional)

- Wooden skewers

Mode of Preparation

1. Thread a cherry tomato, a mozzarella ball, and a basil leaf onto each skewer, repeating until all ingredients are used.

2. Arrange the skewers on a serving platter and drizzle with balsamic glaze if desired.

Nutritional Information

- Calories: 90

- Protein: 6g

- Carbohydrates: 3g

- Fat: 6g

- Fiber: 1g

Serving Size: 2 skewers

Preparation Time: 10 minutes

10: Avocado and Shrimp Cocktail

Health Benefits

- Avocado provides healthy fats and fiber, promoting satiety and digestive health.

- Shrimp is a lean source of protein and omega-3 fatty acids, supporting heart health and muscle function.

- Cocktail sauce adds flavor without adding extra fat or calories.

Ingredients

- 1 ripe avocado, diced

- Peeled and deveined 8 large cooked shrimp.

- Cocktail sauce (store-bought or homemade)

- Fresh lemon wedges for garnish (optional)

Mode of Preparation

1. Divide the diced avocado among serving glasses or small bowls.

2. Top each serving with two cooked shrimp.

3. Drizzle with cocktail sauce and garnish with fresh lemon wedges if desired.

Nutritional Information

- Calories: 120

- Protein: 8g

- Carbohydrates: 5g

- Fat: 8g

- Fiber: 3g

Serving Size: 1 serving

Preparation Time: 10 minutes

<h1 style="text-align:center">CHAPTER 5</h1>

Dessert

1. Berry and Yogurt Parfait

Health Benefits

This parfait is packed with antioxidants from the berries and probiotics from the yogurt, which can help support digestive health and reduce inflammation associated with GERD.

Ingredients

- 1 cup of low-fat Greek yogurt

- Mixed berries of 1/2 cup (such as strawberries, blueberries, and raspberries)

- 1/4 cup of granola (choose low-fat, low-sugar options)

- Honey of 1 tablespoon (optional, for sweetness)

Mode of Preparation

1. In a small bowl or glass, layer the Greek yogurt, mixed berries, and granola.

2. Drizzle honey on top if desired for added sweetness.

3. Repeat layering until all ingredients are used up.

4. It should be served immediately or refrigerate until ready to eat.

Nutritional Information

- Calories: 200

- Protein: 12g

- Carbohydrates: 30g

- Fat: 5g

- Fiber: 4g

- Sugar: 16g

Serving Size: 1 parfait

Preparation Time: 5 minutes

2. Cucumber and Hummus Bites

Health Benefits

Cucumbers are hydrating and low in acid, making them gentle on the stomach. Hummus provides protein and fiber, promoting satiety and aiding in digestion.

Ingredients

- 1 English cucumber

- 1/2 cup of hummus (choose a low-fat, low-sodium variety)

- Fresh dill or parsley for garnish

Mode of Preparation

1. Slice the cucumber into rounds, about 1/4 inch thick.

2. Spoon a small dollop of hummus onto each cucumber slice.

3. Garnish with fresh dill or parsley.

4. Arrange the cucumber and hummus bites on a serving platter and serve immediately.

Nutritional Information

- Calories: 50

- Protein: 3g

- Carbohydrates: 7g

- Fat: 2g

- Fiber: 2g

- Sugar: 1g

Serving Size: 4 bites

Preparation Time: 10 minutes

3. Baked Apple Slices

Health Benefits

Apples are naturally low in acid and high in fiber, making them a soothing choice for GERD patients. Baking them enhances their natural sweetness without adding extra sugar.

Ingredients

- 2 medium apples (such as Granny Smith or Honeycrisp)
- 1 teaspoon of cinnamon
- 1 tablespoon of honey (optional)

Mode of Preparation

1. Preheat the oven to 375°F (190°C).

2. Core the apples and slice them into 1/4-inch thick slices.

3. Place the apple slices on a baking sheet lined with parchment paper.

4. Sprinkle cinnamon evenly over the apple slices.

5. Drizzle honey on top if desired.

6. Bake in the preheated oven for 15-20 minutes, or until the apples are tender.

7. Serve warm or at room temperature.

Nutritional Information

- Calories: 80

- Protein: 0g

- Carbohydrates: 22g

- Fat: 0g

- Fiber: 4g

- Sugar: 16g

Serving Size: 1/2 apple

Cooking Time: 15-20 minutes

Preparation Time: 10 minutes

4. Avocado and Tomato Salad

Health Benefits

Avocados are rich in healthy fats and fiber, which can help soothe the stomach lining. Tomatoes are low in acid and provide vitamins and antioxidants.

Ingredients

- 1 ripe avocado, diced

- 1 cup of cherry tomatoes, halved

- Red onion of 1/4 cup, thinly sliced

- 1 tablespoon of fresh lemon juice

- Salt and pepper to taste

- Fresh basil leaves for garnish

Mode of Preparation

1. In a large bowl, combine the diced avocado, cherry tomatoes, and sliced red onion.

2. Drizzle lemon juice over the salad and gently toss to coat.

3. It should be seasoned Salt and pepper to taste.

4. Fresh basil leaves should be use for garnishing before serving.

Nutritional Information

- Calories: 120

- Protein: 2g

- Carbohydrates: 9g

- Fat: 9g

- Fiber: 5g

- Sugar: 2g

Serving Size: 1 cup

Preparation Time: 10 minutes

5. Chia Seed Pudding

Health Benefits

Chia seeds are rich in fiber and omega-3 fatty acids, which can promote digestive health and reduce inflammation. This pudding is also dairy-free, making it suitable for those with lactose intolerance.

Ingredients

- 2 tablespoons of chia seeds
- 1/2 cup of unsweetened almond milk (or any non-dairy milk of choice)
- 1/2 teaspoon of vanilla extract
- Honey of 1 tablespoon (optional, for sweetness)
- Fresh berries for topping

Mode of Preparation

1. In a small bowl or jar, combine the chia seeds, almond milk, vanilla extract, and honey (if using).
2. Stir well to combine and ensure there are no clumps.

3. Cover the bowl or jar and refrigerate for at least 2
   hours or overnight, until the mixture thickens and
   resembles pudding.

4. Serve chilled, topped with fresh berries.

Nutritional Information

- Calories: 100

- Protein: 3g

- Carbohydrates: 10g

- Fat: 6g

- Fiber: 6g

- Sugar: 2g

Serving Size: 1/2 cup

Preparation Time: 5 minutes (plus chilling time)

6. Grilled Vegetable Skewers

Health Benefits

Grilling vegetables enhances their flavors without adding extra fat, making this dish both tasty and GERD-friendly. Vegetables are also rich in fiber and antioxidants, promoting digestive health.

Ingredients

- 1 zucchini, sliced into rounds

- 1 yellow squash, sliced into rounds

- 1 bell pepper, cut into chunks

- 1 red onion, cut into chunks

- 8 cherry tomatoes

- 2 tablespoons of olive oil

- Dried Italian herbs of 1 teaspoon (such as oregano, basil, and thyme)

- Salt and pepper to taste

- Wooden skewers, soaked in water for at least 30 minutes

Mode of Preparation

1. Preheat the grill to medium-high heat.

2. Thread the vegetables onto the soaked wooden skewers, alternating between different types of vegetables.

3. In a small bowl, whisk together the olive oil, dried Italian herbs, salt, and pepper.

4. Brush the vegetable skewers with the olive oil mixture on all sides.

5. Place the skewers on the preheated grill and cook for 8-10 minutes, turning occasionally, until the vegetables are tender and lightly charred.

6. Skewers should be removed from the grill and serve hot.

Nutritional Information

- Calories: 120

- Protein: 2g

- Carbohydrates: 10g

- Fat: 8g

- Fiber: 3g

- Sugar: 5g

Serving Size: 2 skewers

Cooking Time: 8-10 minutes

Preparation Time: 15 minutes

7. Quinoa Stuffed Bell Peppers
Health Benefits

Quinoa is a nutritious whole grain that is gentle on the stomach and provides protein and fiber. Bell peppers are low in acid and high in vitamins and antioxidants.

Ingredients

- Bell peppers (4) of any color, halved and seeded

- 1 cup of cooked quinoa

- 1 cup of cooked black beans

- 1 cup of diced tomatoes

- 1/2 cup of corn kernels (fresh or frozen)

- 1/4 cup of chopped fresh cilantro

- 1 teaspoon of ground cumin

- 1/2 teaspoon of chili powder

- Salt and pepper to taste

- 1/2 cup of shredded low-fat cheese (optional)

Mode of Preparation

1. Preheat the oven to 375°F (190°C).

2. In a large bowl, combine the cooked quinoa, black beans, diced tomatoes, corn kernels, chopped cilantro, ground cumin, chili powder, salt, and pepper.

3. Spoon the quinoa mixture into the halved bell peppers, dividing it evenly among them.

4. If using cheese, sprinkle it on top of the stuffed peppers.

5. Stuffed peppers should be placed in a baking dish and cover with foil.

6. It should be baked in the preheated oven for 25-30 minutes, or until the peppers are tender.

7. Remove the foil and bake for an additional 5 minutes to melt the cheese (if using).

8. Serve hot, garnished with extra cilantro if desired.

Nutritional Information

- Calories: 200

- Protein: 9g

- Carbohydrates: 35g

- Fat: 3g

- Fiber: 8g

- Sugar: 6g

Serving Size: 1 stuffed pepper half

Cooking Time: 30-35 minutes

Preparation Time: 20 minutes

8. Mango Coconut Chia Seed Pudding

Health Benefits

This tropical-inspired chia seed pudding is rich in fiber and healthy fats from the chia seeds and coconut milk. Mangoes are also low in acid and provide vitamins and antioxidants.

Ingredients

- 2 tablespoons of chia seeds

- 1/2 cup of light coconut milk

- 1/2 cup of unsweetened almond milk (or any non-dairy milk of choice)

- 1/2 teaspoon of vanilla extract

- Honey of 1 tablespoon (optional, for sweetness)

- 1 ripe mango, diced

Mode of Preparation

1. In a small bowl or jar, combine the chia seeds, coconut milk, almond milk, vanilla extract, and honey (if using).

2. Stir well to combine and ensure there are no clumps.

3. Cover the bowl or jar and refrigerate for at least 2 hours or overnight, until the mixture thickens and resembles pudding.

4. In serving glasses or bowls, layer the chia seed pudding with diced mango.

5. Serve chilled and enjoy!

Nutritional Information

- Calories: 180

- Protein: 4g

- Carbohydrates: 25g

- Fat: 8g

- Fiber: 8g

- Sugar: 16g

Serving Size: 1/2 cup of pudding with diced mango

Preparation Time: 5 minutes (plus chilling time)

9. Baked Sweet Potato Fries

Health Benefits

Sweet potatoes are a GERD-friendly alternative to regular potatoes as they are less acidic. They are also rich in fiber, vitamins, and minerals, promoting digestive health.

Ingredients

- 2 medium sweet potatoes, washed and peeled

- 1 tablespoon of olive oil

- 1 teaspoon of smoked paprika

- 1/2 teaspoon of garlic powder

- Salt and pepper to taste

Mode of Preparation

1. Oven should be pre heated to 425°F (220°C) and baking sheet should be line with parchment paper

2. Cut the sweet potatoes into evenly sized fries or wedges.

3. In a large bowl, toss the sweet potato fries with olive oil, smoked paprika, garlic powder, salt, and pepper until well coated.

4. Spread the sweet potato fries in a single layer on the prepared baking sheet, ensuring they are not crowded.

5. Bake in the preheated oven for 20-25 minutes, flipping halfway through, until the fries are golden brown and crispy.

6. It should be removed from the oven and serve hot.

Nutritional Information

- Calories: 120

- Protein: 2g

- Carbohydrates: 20g

- Fat: 4g

- Fiber: 3g

- Sugar: 5g

Serving Size: 1/2 cup of fries

Cooking Time: 20-25 minutes

Preparation Time: 10 minutes

10. Mixed Berry Smoothie Bowl

Health Benefits

This smoothie bowl is packed with antioxidants, fiber, and vitamins from the mixed berries, banana, and spinach, promoting digestive health and reducing inflammation.

Ingredients

- Mixed berries of 1 cup (such as strawberries, blueberries, and raspberries), frozen

- 1 ripe banana, peeled and frozen

- 1/2 cup of baby spinach

- 1/2 cup of unsweetened almond milk (or any non-dairy milk of choice)

- 1 tablespoon of chia seeds

- Toppings: sliced banana, fresh berries, granola, shredded coconut (optional)

Mode of Preparation

1. In a blender, combine the mixed berries, frozen banana, baby spinach, almond milk, and chia seeds.

2. Blend until smooth and creamy, adding more almond milk if needed to reach your desired consistency.

3. Pour the smoothie into a bowl and top with sliced banana, fresh berries, granola, and shredded coconut if desired.

4. Serve immediately and enjoy with a spoon!

Nutritional Information

- Calories: 200

- Protein: 4g

- Carbohydrates: 40g

- Fat: 5g

- Fiber: 8g

- Sugar: 20g

Serving Size: 1 smoothie bowl

Preparation Time: 5 minutes

CHAPTER 6

7 Days Meal Plan

Day 1

Breakfast	Berry and Banana Smoothie
Lunch	Grilled Chicken and Vegetable Salad
Dinner	Baked Salmon with Lemon-Dill Sauce

Day 2

Breakfast	Oatmeal with Almond Butter and Sliced Apples
Lunch	Quinoa and Vegetable Stir-Fry
Dinner	Veggie and Lentil Stuffed Bell Peppers

Day 3

Breakfast	Greek Yogurt Parfait with Granola and Berries
Lunch	Turkey and Avocado Wrap
Dinner	Turkey Meatballs with Zucchini Noodles

Day 4

Breakfast	Scrambled Tofu with Spinach and Tomatoes
Lunch	Lentil Soup with Spinach
Dinner	Vegetable Stir-Fry with Tofu

Day 5

Breakfast	Whole Wheat Toast with Avocado and Sliced Hard-Boiled Eggs
Lunch	Baked Salmon with Steamed Vegetables
Dinner	Vegetable and Lentil Soup

Day 6

Breakfast	Whole Wheat Toast with Avocado and Sliced Hard-Boiled Eggs
Lunch	Turkey and Quinoa Stuffed Bell Peppers
Dinner	Grilled Chicken and Vegetable Skewers

Day 7

Breakfast	Spinach and Feta Egg Muffins
Lunch	Veggie and Hummus Wrap
Dinner	Turkey and Vegetable Stir-Fry with Brown Rice

CHAPTER 7

Conclusion

GERD Diet Cookbook for Seniors is paramount to ascertain the importance of dietary choices in managing Gastroesophageal Reflux Disease (GERD). Throughout this cookbook, we have explored a variety of recipes and meal options specifically tailored to meet the needs of seniors dealing with GERD symptoms. By focusing on gentle, GERD-friendly ingredients and mindful preparation techniques, these recipes aim to alleviate discomfort and promote digestive health.

Managing GERD involves more than just avoiding trigger foods; it requires a holistic approach that encompasses lifestyle modifications, portion control, and mindful eating habits. Through the recipes and guidelines provided in this cookbook, seniors can gain the knowledge and tools necessary to make informed dietary decisions and take control of their digestive well-being.

It is crucial to recognize that each individual may have unique triggers and preferences, and adjustments may be necessary to suit personal tastes and dietary restrictions.

Experimentation and exploration are encouraged, guided by the principles outlined in this cookbook.

As we conclude this journey, let us remember that managing GERD is a continuous process that requires patience, persistence, and self-care. By prioritizing nourishing, GERD-friendly meals and embracing a balanced approach to eating, seniors can enjoy improved quality of life and overall well-being.

May this cookbook serve as a valuable resource and companion on your journey to better digestive health. Here's to delicious meals, good health, and a brighter future ahead.

THANKS FOR READING

9 798888 0276974

THE SIMPLE DIVERTICULITIS COOKBOOK: 2024 Edition

"Nutrition Guide with Delicious Recipes to Comfort and Calm the Gut to Restore Your Health"

Liam Bryce

Table of Contents:

INTRODUCTION

There once was a lively person by the name of Bryce who lived in the busy city of 2024. Bryce was well-known for her indomitable spirit and her love of cooking, but when she was diagnosed with diverticulitis; her devotion was put to the test. She found it challenging to enjoy her favorite foods because of her disease, and she frequently felt lost in the maze of dietary limitations. In the middle of her battle, Bryce came into the "The Simple Diverticulitis Cookbook: 2024 Edition." This book was more than just a cookbook; it was a ray of hope, containing a wide range of dishes that would change eating habits without compromising flavor. Flipping through the pages, Bryce discovered diverticulitis-safe recipes and professional nutritional advice that would hopefully put her culinary adventure back on track. Bryce started a culinary journey with this newfound motivation, embracing vibrant, tasty, and micro biota-friendly plant-based meals that not only satiated her palate but also improved her health. Nutritious dishes designed to control diverticulitis flare-ups, became her go-to friend.

Bryce discovered that as she worked through the recipes, she was able to restore her sense of control over her health in addition to her love of cooking. She was able to enjoy every meal without inducing uncomfortable symptoms thanks to the cookbook's all-natural approach and simple-to-make recipes, which gave her the courage to face the obstacles of Diverticulitis illness. Thanks to the "The Simple Diverticulitis Cookbook: 2024 Edition," Bryce's narrative became one of gastronomic joy and resiliency instead of difficulty. Her experience served as an example of the cookbook's significant influence not just as a manual for handling a medical issue but also as a tribute to the power of delectable, health-promoting cuisine.

Understanding Diverticulitis

A medical illness called diverticulitis is typified by the development of tiny pouches (diverticula) in the walls of the digestive tract, especially in the colon (large intestine). These pouches can become inflamed or infected. Diverticula, or these pouches, are created when weak points in the colon's muscular walls protrude outward. Diverticulitis results from inflammation.

Diverticulitis's precise etiology is unknown; however, a low-fiber diet is frequently linked to it. Constipation can be caused by consuming insufficient amounts of fiber, which can raise intestinal pressure and cause diverticula to develop. Frequent signs and symptoms of diverticulitis include fever, nausea, altered bowel habits, and abdominal pain usually on the left side. Severe instances may result in consequences such as the formation of an abscess, colon perforation, or intestinal obstruction.

Dietary modifications, such as a high-fiber diet to encourage regular bowel movements and avoid constipation, are frequently part of the treatment for diverticulitis. Antibiotics may be recommended in some situations to treat infections, and surgery may be required in more serious or recurrent instances. For an accurate diagnosis and course of treatment, it's critical that those exhibiting symptoms suggestive of diverticulitis get medical assistance. In order to properly treat the illness, healthcare providers may also offer advice on dietary and lifestyle modifications.

Importance of Diet in Managing Symptoms

An important factor in controlling diverticulitis symptoms is diet. The following are some main arguments for the significance of nutrition in the treatment of this condition:

Preventing flare-ups: Diverticulitis symptoms can be aggravated or brought on by specific foods. By adhering to a certain diet, people can lower their chance of flare-ups and the pain and discomfort they cause by avoiding identified trigger foods. Encouraging Regular Bowel Movements: Consuming a diet high in fiber might encourage regular bowel movements. This is crucial for managing diverticulitis since constipation and straining during bowel movements can both cause inflammation and aid in the formation of diverticula.

Minus Inflammation: One of the main characteristics of diverticulitis is inflammation. Certain meals can help lessen inflammation in the digestive tract, relieve symptoms, and encourage recovery. These foods are particularly beneficial when they are high in fiber and have anti-inflammatory qualities.

Managing Symptoms During Flare-Ups: Dietary changes are frequently necessary to reduce the strain on the digestive system when diverticulitis symptoms are severe. A well-thought-out diet may offer nourishment while steering clear of items that could exacerbate inflammation.

Supporting Gut Health: For people with diverticulitis, maintaining a healthy gut is essential. Eating a well-balanced diet helps. Probiotics and fermented foods are two examples of foods that can help the digestive system and encourage a healthy balance of gut flora.

Avoiding Complications: Eating a healthy diet will help avoid diverticulitis-related problems such as intestinal obstruction, perforation, and abscess development. This is especially crucial for people who have experienced severe or recurring diverticulitis in the past.

Enhancing Nutrient Absorption: Eating a balanced diet guarantees that people get the important nutrients they need, which promotes general health. Sufficient nourishment is crucial for the body's capacity to mend and rebound, particularly during and following bouts of diverticulitis.

Improving Quality of Life: People with diverticulitis can have a higher quality of life overall by properly controlling their food. This entails easing the symptoms, lessening the severity of flare-ups, and fostering wellbeing.

It's crucial to remember that each person may require different food suggestions depending on their unique medical history, level of symptoms, and other factors. Creating a customized and successful food plan for controlling diverticulitis requires speaking with a medical expert or a qualified dietitian.

DIETARY GUIDELINES

High-Fiber Foods for Digestive Health

High-fiber foods are essential for maintaining digestive health, and they play a significant role in managing conditions like diverticulitis. Here is a list of high-fiber foods that are beneficial for digestive health:

Whole Grains:

- Brown rice
- Quinoa Oats (steel-cut or old-fashioned)
- Whole-wheat pasta
- Barley

Legumes:

- Lentils
- Chickpeas
  Black beans
- Kidney beans

- Split peas

Vegetables

- Broccoli

- Brussels sprouts

- Carrots

- Spinach

- Kale

- Sweet potatoes

Fruits:

- Apples (with the skin)

- Pears

- Berries (strawberries, blueberries, and raspberries)

- Oranges

- Bananas

Nuts and Seeds:

- Almonds

- Chia seeds

- Flaxseeds

- Sunflower seeds

- Walnuts

Whole Grain Cereals:

Bran flakes

Whole-grain cereal (check for low sugar content)

Muesli

Bread and Tortillas:

- Whole-grain bread

- Whole-wheat tortillas

- Rye bread

Dried Fruits:

- Prunes
- Figs
- Apricots

Popcorn: Air-popped popcorn is a good source of fiber, but it's important to consume it in moderation and without excessive butter or oil.

High-Fiber Snacks:

Raw vegetables with hummus

Trail mix with nuts and dried fruits unsweetened Greek yogurt with added fiber (check labels)

Including a variety of these high-fiber foods in your diet can contribute to better digestive health. In addition to promoting regular bowel movements and a healthy gut environment, fiber also helps avoid constipation., and supports a healthy gut environment. However, for individuals with diverticulitis or other digestive conditions, it's essential to introduce fiber gradually to avoid potential discomfort, and consulting with a healthcare professional or a registered dietitian is advisable to create a personalized dietary plan.

Low-Residue Diet Explained

A low-residue diet is a dietary approach that restricts the intake of foods that are high in fiber and other indigestible materials. The term "residue" refers to the undigested or partially digested food that makes its way through the digestive system and is eventually eliminated as stool. This type of diet is often recommended for individuals with certain medical conditions, including diverticulitis, inflammatory bowel disease (IBD), or before certain medical procedures like colonoscopies. Here's an explanation of the key principles of a low-residue diet:

Low-Fiber Foods:

The main focus of a low-residue diet is to limit the consumption of high-fiber foods. This includes avoiding whole grains, bran, seeds, nuts, and raw fruits and vegetables.

Refined Grains:

White bread, white rice, and refined pasta are generally allowed on a low-residue diet. These are easier to digest compared to their whole-grain counterparts.

Well-Cooked Vegetables:

Some well-cooked and peeled vegetables may be permitted, but typically in limited quantities. Examples include peeled and cooked potatoes, carrots, and green beans.

Fruit Juices and Peeled Fruits:

Fruit juices without pulp and peeled fruits (such as apples without skin) are often included, while high-fiber fruits with seeds are restricted.

Limited Dairy:

Dairy products are usually allowed, but individuals may need to limit their intake of high-lactose items if lactose intolerance is a concern.

Lean Proteins:

Lean proteins, such as poultry, fish, eggs, and well-cooked tender meats, are generally well-tolerated on a low-residue diet.

Processed Foods:

Some processed foods, like cereals and snacks made with refined grains, may be suitable for a low-residue diet, but it's essential to check labels for added fiber.

The goal of a low-residue diet is to reduce the bulk and frequency of bowel movements, provide the digestive system with a break, and minimize irritation to the intestines. This can be particularly helpful during periods of inflammation or after surgery. However, it's important to note that a low-residue diet is usually a temporary measure, and individuals should transition back to a more balanced and varied diet under the guidance of a healthcare professional.

As with any dietary changes, it's crucial for individuals to consult with their healthcare team, including a registered dietitian, to ensure that their nutritional needs are met while adhering to the requirements of a low-residue diet

Foods to Avoid and Alternatives

In managing diverticulitis, there are certain foods that individuals are often advised to avoid to prevent irritation and reduce the risk of flare-ups. Here's a list of foods to avoid and potential alternatives that may be more suitable for individuals with diverticulitis: Foods to Avoid:

Nuts and Seeds:

Avoid:

Whole nuts and seeds

Alternative: Nut and seed butters (smooth varieties without added seeds)

Popcorn:

Avoid: Regular popcorn

Alternative: Puffed rice or other low-fiber snacks

Whole Grains with High Fiber:

Avoid: Whole wheat bread, brown rice, and whole grain cereals.

Alternative: White bread, white rice, refined cereals

Certain Raw Fruits and Vegetables:

Avoid: Raw apples, raw carrots, broccoli, cauliflower
Alternative: Cooked or peeled fruits and well-cooked vegetables

Tough Skins and Fibrous Parts:

Avoid: Tough meat with gristle, sausage casings
Alternative: Tender meats, poultry without skin, lean fish

Beans and Legumes:

Avoid: Beans, lentils, and chickpeas
Alternative: well-cooked and peeled legumes in moderation

High-Fiber Snacks:

Avoid: Trail mix with nuts and seeds, high-fiber bars
Alternative: Low-fiber snacks, such as crackers or pretzels

Dried Fruits:

Avoid: Raisins, dried apricots, and prunes.
Alternative: Fresh or canned fruits (without added sugar), in moderation.

Spicy Foods:

Avoid Spicy and hot foods that may irritate the digestive tract

Alternative: Mildly seasoned dishes without excessive spice

Certain Dairy Products:

Avoid High-lactose dairy if lactose intolerant. Alternative: Lactose-free or low-lactose dairy options It's important to note that the severity of diverticulitis can vary among individuals, and dietary recommendations may be personalized based on specific symptoms and medical advice. Additionally, reintroducing avoided foods should be done gradually to assess individual tolerance

KITCHEN TIPS FOR DIGESTIVE WELLNESS

Gentle Cooking Techniques

Incorporating gentle cooking techniques is key to creating flavorful and easily digestible meals. Here are some recommended gentle cooking techniques that can be highlighted in the cookbook:

Steaming:

Steaming is a gentle cooking method that helps retain the nutritional value of vegetables while making them softer and easier to digest. Include recipes for steamed broccoli, cauliflower, and other veggies.

Poaching:

Poaching involves gently simmering food in liquid, often with added herbs and spices. This technique is suitable for cooking lean proteins like chicken or fish, keeping them moist and tender.

Baking:

Baking is a versatile method that can be used for proteins, vegetables, and grains. It allows for gentle cooking without excessive heat, resulting in flavorful and easily digestible dishes.

Slow Cooking:

Slow cooking in a crockpot or slow cooker is ideal for tenderizing tougher cuts of meat and creating savory stews or soups. This method allows flavors to meld while keeping the ingredients soft.

Pressure Cooking:

Pressure cooking can be used to cook grains, legumes, and meats quickly while maintaining their tenderness. It's a time-efficient way to prepare meals without compromising on texture.

Sautéing with Care:

Sautéing vegetables or proteins with minimal oil over low to medium heat is a gentle way to add flavor without excessive browning. This technique preserves the texture and nutritional content of the ingredients.

Blanching:

Blanching involves briefly immersing vegetables in boiling water and then quickly cooling them. This technique helps to soften vegetables while preserving their vibrant colors and nutrients.

Mashing and pureeing:

For individuals who may have difficulty with certain textures, recipes that involve mashing or pureeing can be included. This is especially useful for incorporating vegetables into soups or creating smooth, textured side dishes.

Grilling with Caution:

Grilling can add a smoky flavor to food, but it's essential to do it with caution. Choose lean cuts of meat and vegetables and avoid excessive charring, as high temperatures and burned parts may be harsh on the digestive system.

One-Pot Meals:

Creating one-pot meals simplifies the cooking process and minimizes the need for excessive handling. Recipes like casseroles or slow-cooked stews can be featured in the cookbook.

Recommended Utensils and Equipment

Recommending the right utensils and equipment can make the cooking process more accessible and enjoyable for individuals managing diverticulitis. Here are some recommended utensils and equipment for the cookbook:

Steamer Basket:

A steamer basket is useful for gently cooking vegetables, preserving their nutritional value while making them soft and easy to digest.

Slow Cooker or Crockpot:

These appliances are convenient for slow-cooking meats, stews, and soups, allowing for tender and flavorful dishes without excessive handling.

Blender or Food Processor:

These appliances are essential for pureeing or blending ingredients, creating smooth textures suitable for those who prefer or require softer foods.

Non-Stick Cookware:

Non-stick pans and pots minimize the need for excessive oil or fat during cooking, making it easier to prepare meals with a lower fat content.

Pressure Cooker:

A pressure cooker is efficient for cooking grains, legumes, and meats quickly, maintaining tenderness without prolonged cooking times.

Baking Sheets and Pans:

These are versatile for baking lean proteins, vegetables, and grains. They allow for gentle cooking and can be used for one-pan meals.

Chef's Knife and Cutting Board:

A sharp chef's knife and a stable cutting board are fundamental for safe and efficient meal preparation.

Slow Juicer:

For individuals who enjoy fresh juices, a slow juicer is a gentle way to extract juice without generating excess heat, which may affect nutrient content.

Strainer or Colander:

These are useful for draining and rinsing ingredients, particularly for recipes involving canned beans or pasta.

Mortar and Pestle:

For grinding herbs and spices, a mortar and pestle provide a gentle method that enhances flavor without relying on pre-packaged spice blends.

Measuring Cups and Spoons:

Accurate measurements are crucial in cooking, especially for individuals following specific dietary recommendations. Measuring cups and spoons ensure precision.

Silicone or Wooden Utensils:

Non-abrasive utensils like silicone or wooden spatulas and spoons are gentle on cookware and can be used for stirring and serving.

Cutting Scissors:

Scissors designed for cutting herbs or small ingredients directly into a dish can be a helpful addition.

Food Thermometer:

For ensuring meats are cooked to the right temperature without overcooking, a food thermometer is a handy tool.

Including information about these utensils and equipment in the cookbook helps individuals with diverticulitis prepare meals more easily and promotes a positive cooking experience

Portion Control

Portion control is a crucial aspect of managing diverticulitis and promoting digestive health. In the "Simple Diverticulitis Cookbook: 2024 Edition," incorporating guidance on portion control can help individuals enjoy balanced meals without overloading their digestive system. Here are some tips on portion control that can be emphasized in the cookbook:

Serve Smaller Portions:

Encourage smaller serving sizes to avoid overwhelming the digestive tract. Providing recipes with predetermined serving sizes can guide individuals in managing their portions effectively.

Use smaller Plates:

Opting for smaller plates creates an optical illusion, making portions appear larger. This psychological trick can help individuals feel satisfied with smaller amounts of food.

Include a Variety of Foods:

Design recipes that include a variety of nutrient-dense foods to ensure that individuals get a well-rounded meal, even with smaller portions. This promotes overall nutritional balance.

Emphasize Quality Over Quantity:

Focus on the quality of ingredients and flavors rather than the quantity of food. Encourage savoring each bite, promoting mindful eating and satisfaction with smaller portions.

Provide Clear Serving Sizes:

Clearly indicate the intended serving sizes for each recipe in the cookbook. This helps individuals follow dietary recommendations and avoid excessive consumption.

Balanced Meal Composition:

Design recipes that balance protein, carbohydrates, and healthy fats to create satisfying meals without the need for large portions.

Encourage Regular, Small Meals:

Suggest eating smaller meals throughout the day rather than a few large ones. This approach can help maintain energy levels and prevent overeating during main meals.

Mindful Eating Practices:

Promote mindfulness during meals by encouraging individuals to eat slowly, chew thoroughly, and pay attention to hunger and fullness cues. Mindful eating supports better portion control.

Offer Snack Ideas:

Include snack options in the cookbook with portion-controlled suggestions. This helps individuals manage hunger between meals without resorting to large snacks.

Incorporate Visual Guides:

Use visual guides, such as images or illustrations, to demonstrate appropriate portion sizes. This can be particularly helpful for individuals who are learning about portion control.

Consult with Healthcare Professionals:

Recommend that individuals consult with their healthcare provider or a registered dietitian to determine personalized portion sizes based on their specific health needs and dietary requirements.

BEVERAGES FOR HYDRATION

Infused Water Recipes

Infused water can be a delightful and hydrating addition to the "Simple Diverticulitis Cookbook: 2024 Edition." These infused water recipes provide a burst of natural flavors without the need for added sugars or artificial ingredients. Here are some refreshing infused water recipes to consider:

Citrus Mint Infusion

Ingredients:

- 1 lemon (sliced)
- 1 lime (sliced)
- 1 orange (sliced)
- Fresh mint leaves
- Ice cubes

Instructions:

Combine lemon slices, lime slices, orange slices, and a handful of fresh mint leaves in a pitcher. Add ice cubes to the pitcher. Fill the pitcher with water and let it sit in the refrigerator for at least an hour to allow the flavors to infuse.

Pour over ice and enjoy the citrusy freshness.

Berry Basil Bliss

Ingredients:

- 1 cup mixed berries (strawberries, blueberries, raspberries)
- Fresh basil leaves
- Ice cubes

Instructions:

In a pitcher, mix the mixed berries and a handful of fresh basil leaves.

Add ice cubes to the pitcher.

Fill the pitcher with water and refrigerate for a couple of hours to let the flavors meld. Serve over ice for a Delightful berry- and basil-infused drink.

Cucumber Rosemary Refresher

Ingredients:

- 1/2 cucumber (sliced)
- Fresh rosemary sprigs
- Ice cubes

Instructions:

Place cucumber slices and fresh rosemary sprigs in a pitcher.

Add ice cubes to the pitcher.

Fill the pitcher with water and let it infuse in the refrigerator for a few hours.

Pour over ice for a crisp and refreshing cucumber rhizome infusion.

Pineapple Coconut Paradise

Ingredients:

- 1 cup of pineapple chunks
- Coconut water
- Ice cubes

Instructions:

Add pineapple chunks to a pitcher.

Fill the pitcher with coconut water.

Add ice cubes to enhance the chill factor.

Allow the mixture to infuse for a few hours before serving over ice for a tropical paradise experience.

Apple Cinnamon Spice

Ingredients:

- 1 apple (sliced)
- Cinnamon sticks
- Ice cubes

Instructions:

Mix apple slices and cinnamon sticks in a pitcher.

Add ice cubes to the pitcher.

Fill the pitcher with water and refrigerate for a few hours to let the apple and cinnamon flavors meld. Serve over ice for lightly sweet and spice-infused water.

These infused water recipes offer a tasty and hydrating alternative to sugary beverages, making them a delightful addition to the "Simple

Diverticulitis Cookbook." They provide a burst of natural flavors without compromising digestive health.

Herbal Teas for Soothing the Digestive Tract

There are two recipes for herbal teas that may help in calming and supporting digestion:

Peppermint Digestive Tea:

Ingredients:

- 1 peppermint tea bag or 1 tablespoon dried peppermint leaves

- 1 teaspoon fennel seeds

- 1 teaspoon chamomile flowers (optional)

- Honey or lemon for taste (optional)

Instructions:

Boil Water:

Boiling cup of water to boiling point.

Prepare Tea Infusion:

Place the peppermint tea bag, fennel seeds, and chamomile flowers (if using) in a cup.

Pour Hot Water:

Pour the hot water over the ingredients in the cup.

Steep:

Let the tea steep for 5-7 minutes to allow the flavors to infuse.

Strain (if necessary):

If you used loose peppermint leaves and chamomile flowers, strain the tea to remove the herbs.

Add Sweetener (Optional):

Add honey or lemon for a touch of sweetness if desired.

Enjoy:

Sip and enjoy this soothing peppermint digestive tea after meals or whenever you need a calming moment.

Ginger-Lemon Digestive Tea:

Ingredients:

- 1 inch fresh ginger, sliced

- 1 tablespoon dried chamomile flowers

- 1 tablespoon dried lemon balm leaves (or a few slices of fresh lemon)

- Honey for taste (optional)

Instructions:

Boil Water:

Boiling cup of water to boiling point.

Prepare Tea Infusion:

Place the fresh ginger slices, chamomile flowers, and lemon balm leaves (or fresh lemon slices) in a cup.

Pour Hot Water:

Pour the hot water over the ingredients in the cup.

Steep:

Let the tea steep for 5-7 minutes to allow the flavors to meld.

Strain (if necessary):

If you used loose herbs, strain the tea to remove the ginger and herbs.

Add Sweetener (Optional):

Add honey for a touch of sweetness if like.

Enjoy:

Sip on this invigorating ginger-lemon digestive tea to aid digestion and provide a comforting sensation.

These herbal teas are not only delicious but also have properties that may help ease digestive discomfort. As with any herbal remedy, if you have specific health concerns or are pregnant, it's advisable to consult with a healthcare professional before incorporating new herbs into your routine.

BREAKFAST DELIGHTS

Fiber-Rich Smoothies

Fiber-rich smoothies are a great way to offer delicious and nutritious options for individuals managing diverticulitis. Here are some fiber-rich smoothie recipes:

Mixed Berry and Spinach Smoothie:

Ingredients:

- 1 cup mixed berries (strawberries, blueberries, raspberries)

- 1/2 banana (ripe)

- 1 cup of fresh spinach leaves

- 1 tablespoon of chia seeds

- 1/2 cup Greek yogurt (low-fat)

- 1 cup water or almond milk (unsweetened)

- Ice cubes (optional)

Instructions:

Blend mixed berries, banana, spinach, chia seeds, Greek yogurt, and water or almond milk until smooth.

Add ice cubes if desired and blend well

Pour into a glass and enjoy the fiber-packed goodness.

Tropical Fiber Boost Smoothie:

Ingredients:

- 1/2 cup pineapple chunks (fresh or frozen)

- 1/2 mango (peeled and diced)

- 1/2 kiwi (peeled and sliced)

- 1 tablespoon flaxseeds

- 1/2 cup Greek yogurt (low-fat)

- 1 cup of coconut water

- Ice cubes (optional)

Instructions:

Blend pineapple, mango, kiwi, flaxseeds, Greek yogurt, and coconut water until smooth.

Add ice cubes if desired and blend well

Pour into a glass and enjoy this tropical fiber boost.

Green Apple and Kale Smoothie:

Ingredients:

- 1 green apple (cored and sliced)

- 1 cup kale leaves (stems removed)

- 1/2 cucumber (peeled and sliced)

- 1 tablespoon of hemp seeds

- 1/2 lemon (juiced)

- 1 cup of water or green tea (unsweetened)

- Ice cubes (optional)

Instructions:

Blend green apple, kale, cucumber, hemp seeds, lemon juice, and water/green tea until well combined.

Add ice cubes if desired and blend well.

Pour into a glass and savor the green apple and kale freshness.

Banana-Oat Power Smoothie:

Ingredients:

- 1 ripe banana

- 1/2 cup rolled oats

- 1 tablespoon of almond butter

- 1/2 cup Greek yogurt (low-fat)

- 1/2 teaspoon cinnamon

- 1 cup almond milk (unsweetened)

- Ice cubes (optional)

Instructions:

Blend banana, oats, almond butter, Greek yogurt, cinnamon, and almond milk until creamy.

Add ice cubes if desired and blend well

Pour into a glass and relish the power-packed banana-oat goodness.

Berry and Avocado Delight:

Ingredients:

- 1 cup mixed berries (strawberries, blueberries, raspberries)

- 1/2 avocado

- 1 tablespoon of chia seeds

- 1/2 cup Greek yogurt (low-fat)

- 1 cup of water or coconut water

- Ice cubes (optional)

Instructions:

Blend mixed berries, avocado, chia seeds, Greek yogurt, and water or coconut water until smooth.

Add ice cubes if desired and blend well

Pour into a glass and enjoy the delightful combination of berries and creamy avocado.

These fiber-rich smoothie recipes provide a tasty and convenient way to incorporate essential nutrients into the diet while considering the dietary needs of individuals managing diverticulitis.

Oatmeal Variations

Including a variety of oatmeal can offer individuals managing diverticulitis a comforting and nutritious breakfast choice. Here are some oatmeal variations to consider:

Classic Cinnamon Apple Oatmeal:

Ingredients:

- 1/2 cup old-fashioned rolled oats
- 1 cup water (dairy or plant-based)
- 1 apple, peeled and diced
- 1/2 teaspoon ground cinnamon

- 1 tablespoon honey or maple syrup (optional)

Instructions:

Cook the oats according to package instructions with water or milk.

Add diced apples and ground cinnamon to the cooking oats.

Stir well, and let the apples soften.

Sweeten with honey, if desired.

Berry Almond Crunch Oatmeal:

Ingredients:

- 1/2 cup old-fashioned rolled oats
- 1 cup of water or almond milk
- 1/2 cup mixed berries (strawberries, blueberries, raspberries)
- 1 tablespoon of almond butter

- 1 tablespoon sliced almonds
- 1 teaspoon of chia seeds

Instructions:

Cook oats in water or almond milk according to package instructions.

Stir in mixed berries, almond butter, sliced almonds, and chia seeds.

Mix well until the berries release their juices and the almond butter is melted.

Pumpkin Spice Pecan Oatmeal:

Ingredients:

- 1/2 cup old-fashioned rolled oats
- 1 cup water (dairy or plant-based)
- 2 tablespoons canned pumpkin puree
- 1/2 teaspoon pumpkin spice
- 1 tablespoon chopped pecans

- 1 tablespoon of maple syrup

Instructions:

Cook oats in water or milk according to package instructions.

Stir in pumpkin puree and pumpkin spice.

Top with chopped pecans, and drizzle with maple syrup.

Banana Nut Oatmeal:

Ingredients:

- 1/2 cup old-fashioned rolled oats
- 1 cup water (dairy or plant-based)
- 1 ripe banana, mashed
- 1 tablespoon chopped walnuts or almonds
- 1/2 teaspoon vanilla extract
- 1 tablespoon honey or agave syrup (optional)

Instructions:

Cook oats in water or milk according to package instructions.

Stir in mashed banana, chopped nuts, and vanilla extract, and sweeten with honey or agave syrup if desired.

Coconut Mango Oatmeal:

Ingredients:

- 1/2 cup old-fashioned rolled oats
- 1 cup of coconut milk
- 1/2 cup diced mango
- 1 tablespoon shredded coconut
- 1 tablespoon chopped macadamia nuts
- 1 teaspoon honey or agave syrup (optional)

Instructions:

Cook oats in coconut milk according to package instructions.

Stir in diced mango, shredded coconut, and chopped macadamia nuts.

Sweeten with honey or agave syrup, if desired.

Blueberry Lemon Chia Oatmeal:

Ingredients:

- 1/2 cup old-fashioned rolled oats
- 1 cup of water or almond milk
- 1/2 cup of fresh or frozen blueberries
- 1 tablespoon of chia seeds
- Zest of one lemon
- 1 tablespoon honey

Instructions:

Cook oats in water or almond milk according to package instructions.

Stir in blueberries, chia seeds, and lemon zest.

Sweeten with honey, if desired.

Chocolate Banana Walnut Oatmeal:

Ingredients:

- 1/2 cup old-fashioned rolled oats
- 1 cup of milk of your choice
- 1 ripe banana, mashed
- 1 tablespoon cocoa powder
- 1 tablespoon chopped walnuts
- 1/2 teaspoon vanilla extract

Instructions:

Cook oats in milk according to package instructions.

Stir in mashed banana, cocoa powder, chopped walnuts, and vanilla extract.

Enjoy the delightful combination of chocolate, banana, and nuts.

Savory Herb and Vegetable Oatmeal:

Ingredients:

- 1/2 cup old-fashioned rolled oats
- 1 cup of vegetable broth
- 1/4 cup diced bell peppers
- 1/4 cup diced tomatoes
- 1 tablespoon chopped fresh herbs (parsley, chives)
- Salt and pepper to taste
- Optional: grated Parmesan cheese

Instructions:

Cook oats in vegetable broth according to package instructions.

Stir in diced bell peppers, diced tomatoes, and fresh herbs.

Season with salt and pepper. Top with grated Parmesan if desired.

Peach Ginger Oatmeal:

Ingredients:

- 1/2 cup old-fashioned rolled oats
- 1 cup of water or coconut milk
- 1 ripe peach, sliced
- 1 teaspoon grated fresh ginger
- 1 tablespoon shredded coconut
- 1 tablespoon slivered almonds
- 1 teaspoon honey

Instructions:

Cook oats in water or coconut milk according to package instructions.

Stir in sliced peaches, grated ginger, shredded coconut, and slivered almonds.

Drizzle with honey, if desired.

Mediterranean-Inspired Savory Oatmeal:

Ingredients:

- 1/2 cup old-fashioned rolled oats
- 1 cup of vegetable broth
- 2 tablespoons diced Kalamata olives
- 1 tablespoon crumbled feta cheese
- 1 tablespoon chopped fresh basil
- 1 tablespoon sun-dried tomatoes, chopped
- Salt and pepper to taste

Instructions:

Cook oats in vegetable broth according to package instructions.

Stir in Kalamata olives, crumbled feta, chopped basil, and sun-dried tomatoes.

Season with salt and pepper for a savory twist on oatmeal.

These oatmeal variations provide a range of flavors, from sweet to savory, ensuring a diverse and satisfying breakfast experience for individuals managing diverticulitis.

Low-Residue Breakfast Options

Egg and Spinach Scramble:

Ingredients:

- Scrambled eggs

- Sautéed spinach
- Salt and pepper to taste

Instructions:

- Cook scrambled eggs.
- Sauté the spinach separately and fold it into the scrambled eggs.
- Season with salt and pepper.

Yogurt Parfait:

Ingredients:

- Low-fiber yogurt
- Soft fruits (peeled and diced bananas or canned peaches)
- Granola

Instructions:

Layer low-fiber yogurt with soft fruits in a glass.

Top with a sprinkle of granola.

Creamy Oatmeal:

Ingredients:

- Well-cooked rolled oats
- Milk
- Nut butter or ground cinnamon for flavor

Instructions:

Cook rolled oats with milk until creamy.

Top with a dollop of nut butter or a sprinkle of ground cinnamon.

Smoothies:

Ingredients:

- Low-fiber fruits (berries, bananas, and melon)
- Yogurt or lactose-free milk

Instructions:

Blend low-fiber fruits with yogurt or lactose-free milk for a refreshing smoothie.

Low-Fiber Pancakes:

Ingredients:

- Pancakes made with refined flour

- Mashed bananas for natural sweetness

- Syrup (in moderation)

Instructions:

Make pancakes using refined flour.

Add mashed bananas to the batter.

Serve with a small amount of syrup.

Soft Scrambled Tofu:

Ingredients:

- Tofu
- Seasonings of choice

Instructions:

Cook tofu with your preferred seasonings until soft.

Scramble and serve as a plant-based alternative to eggs.

Applesauce with Cottage Cheese:

Ingredients:

- Unsweetened applesauce
- Cottage cheese

Instructions:

Combine unsweetened applesauce with cottage cheese for a soft and satisfying breakfast.

Peanut Butter Banana Toast:

Ingredients:

- Toasted white bread
- Peanut butter
- Sliced bananas

Instructions:

Toast white bread.

Spread peanut butter on top and add sliced bananas.

Poached Eggs with White Rice:

Ingredients:

- Poached eggs
- Well-cooked white rice

Instructions:

Poach eggs and serve over well-cooked white rice.

Chia Pudding:

Ingredients:

- Chia seeds
- Lactose-free milk
- Soft fruits (berries, kiwi) for topping

Instructions:

Mix chia seeds with lactose-free milk and let it sit overnight.

Top with soft fruits before serving.

These low-residue breakfast options aim to minimize fiber intake while providing essential nutrients and flavors.

Classic Grilled Chicken Caesar Salad:

Grilled Chicken Salads

Ingredients:

- Grilled chicken breast
- Romaine lettuce, chopped
- Caesar dressing
- Croutons

Parmesan cheese, grated

Instructions:

- Grill a chicken breast and slice it.
- Toss chopped romaine lettuce with Caesar dressing.
- Top with grilled chicken slices, croutons, and grated Parmesan cheese.

Mango Avocado Grilled Chicken Salad:

Ingredients:

- Grilled chicken strips
- Mixed greens
- Diced mango
- Avocado, sliced
- Red onion, thinly sliced
- Mango vinaigrette

Instructions:

Grill chicken strips and let them cool.

In a bowl, combine mixed greens, diced mango, sliced avocado, and thinly sliced red onion.

Add grilled chicken and drizzle with mango vinaigrette.

Greek Grilled Chicken Salad:

Ingredients:

- Grilled chicken chunks
- Cherry tomatoes, halved
- Cucumber, diced
- Kalamata olives, sliced
- Feta cheese, crumbled

- Greek dressing

Instructions:

Grill chicken chunks and set aside.

Mix cherry tomatoes, cucumber, Kalamata olives, and feta cheese in a bowl.

Add the grilled chicken and toss with Greek dressing.

Strawberry Spinach Grilled Chicken Salad:

Ingredients:

- Grilled chicken breast, sliced
- Baby spinach
- Fresh strawberries, sliced
- Goat cheese, crumbled
- Balsamic vinaigrette

Instructions:

Grill a chicken breast and slice it.

In a bowl, combine baby spinach, sliced strawberries, and crumbled goat cheese.

Top with grilled chicken slices and drizzle with balsamic vinaigrette.

Tex-Mex Grilled Chicken Salad:

Ingredients:

- Grilled chicken strips
- Black beans, drained and rinsed
- Corn kernels
- Cherry tomatoes, halved
- Avocado, diced
- Lime-cilantro dressing

Instructions:

Grill chicken strips and set aside.

Mix black beans, corn kernels, cherry tomatoes, and diced avocado in a bowl.

Add grilled chicken and toss with lime-cilantro dressing.

Caprese Grilled Chicken Salad:

Ingredients:

- Grilled chicken breast
- Cherry tomatoes, halved
- Fresh mozzarella, diced
- Basil leaves, torn
- Balsamic glaze

Instructions:

Grill a chicken breast and slice it.

Combine cherry tomatoes, fresh mozzarella, and torn basil leaves in a bowl.

Top with grilled chicken slices and drizzle with balsamic glaze.

Avocado Chickpea Grilled Chicken Salad:

Ingredients:

- Grilled chicken chunks
- Mixed greens
- Avocado, sliced
- Chickpeas, drained and rinsed

- Cherry tomatoes, halved

Lemon-tahini dressing

Instructions:

Grill chicken chunks and let them cool.

Toss mixed greens with sliced avocado, chickpeas, and cherry tomatoes.

Add grilled chicken and drizzle with lemon-tahini dressing.

Salmon and Cream Cheese Grilled Chicken Salad:

Ingredients:

- Grilled chicken strips
- Smoked salmon
- Cream cheese, softened
- Cucumber, thinly sliced
- Dill, chopped

Instructions:

Grill chicken strips and set aside.

In a bowl, mix smoked salmon with softened cream cheese.

Arrange the grilled chicken on a plate with cucumber slices and top with the salmon-cream cheese mixture.

Sprinkle with chopped dill.

Mediterranean Quinoa Grilled Chicken Salad:

Ingredients:

- Grilled chicken breast, sliced
- Quinoa, cooked
- Cherry tomatoes, halved
- Cucumber, diced
- Feta cheese, crumbled
- Kalamata olives, sliced
- Greek dressing

Instructions:

Grill a chicken breast and slice it.

In a bowl, combine cooked quinoa, cherry tomatoes, diced cucumber, feta cheese, and Kalamata olives.

Top with grilled chicken slices, and toss with Greek dressing.

Harvest Grilled Chicken Salad:

Ingredients:

- Grilled chicken chunks
- Mixed greens
- Roasted butternut squash, diced
- Pecans, chopped
- Dried cranberries
- Maple Dijon vinaigrette

Instructions:

Grill chicken chunks and let them cool.

Toss mixed greens with diced roasted butternut squash, chopped pecans, and dried cranberries.

Add grilled chicken and drizzle with maple Dijon vinaigrette.

These grilled chicken salad recipes offer a variety of flavors and textures while considering the dietary needs of individuals managing diverticulitis. Feel free to customize them based on personal preferences and dietary requirements.

LUNCHTIME FAVORITES

Quinoa and Vegetable Bowls

Mediterranean Quinoa Bowl:

Ingredients:

- Cooked quinoa

- Cherry tomatoes, halved

- Cucumber, diced

- Kalamata olives, sliced

- Feta cheese, crumbled

- Fresh lemon juice

- Olive oil

- Fresh oregano, chopped

- Salt and pepper to taste

Instructions:

In a bowl, combine cooked quinoa, cherry tomatoes, cucumber, Kalamata olives, and crumbled feta cheese.

Drizzle with olive oil and fresh lemon juice.

Add chopped fresh oregano and season with salt and pepper.

Toss the ingredients until well combined.

Serve in bowls and enjoy!

Roasted Vegetable Quinoa Bowl:

Ingredients:

- Cooked quinoa

- Bell peppers, sliced

- Zucchini, sliced

- Cherry tomatoes

- Red onion, thinly sliced

- Balsamic glaze

- Olive oil

- Fresh basil, chopped

- Salt and pepper to taste

Instructions:

Preheat the oven to 400°F (200°C).

Toss sliced bell peppers, zucchini, cherry tomatoes, and red onion with olive oil, salt, and pepper.

Roast the vegetables in the oven until they are tender and slightly caramelized.

In a bowl, combine the cooked quinoa with the roasted vegetables.

Drizzle with balsamic glaze and sprinkle with chopped fresh basil.

Mix well, and serve in bowls.

Southwest Quinoa Bowl:

Ingredients:

- Cooked quinoa

- Black beans, drained and rinsed

- Corn kernels (fresh or frozen)

- Cherry tomatoes, halved

- Avocado, diced

- Lime-cilantro dressing

- Fresh cilantro, chopped

- Salt and pepper to taste

Instructions:

In a bowl, combine cooked quinoa, black beans, corn kernels, cherry tomatoes, and diced avocado.

Drizzle with lime-cilantro dressing.

Add chopped fresh cilantro and season with salt and pepper.

Toss the ingredients until well coated with the dressing.

Serve in bowls and enjoy the Southwest flavors!

Asian Sesame Quinoa Bowl:

Ingredients:

- Cooked quinoa

- Stir-fried broccoli, snap peas, and carrots

- Grilled chicken strips

- Sesame seeds

- Soy sauce or tamari

- Sesame oil

- Green onions, sliced

Instructions:

In a bowl, combine cooked quinoa, stir-fried vegetables, and grilled chicken strips.

Drizzle with soy sauce or tamari and sesame oil to taste.

Add chopped green onions and sesame seeds on the top.

Toss the ingredients until well combined.

Serve in bowls for an Asian-inspired delight.

Caprese Quinoa Bowl:

Ingredients:

- Cooked quinoa

- Fresh mozzarella, diced

- Cherry tomatoes, halved

- Basil leaves, torn

- Balsamic glaze

- Olive oil

- Salt and pepper to taste

Instructions:

Mix cooked quinoa with diced fresh mozzarella, cherry tomatoes, and torn basil leaves in a bowl.

Drizzle with a balsamic glaze and olive oil.

Season with salt and pepper, to taste.

Gently toss the ingredients until well coated.

Serve in bowls for a refreshing Caprese experience.

Mango Avocado Quinoa Bowl:

Ingredients:

- Cooked quinoa
- Grilled chicken strips
- Diced mango
- Avocado, diced
- Red onion, finely chopped
- Cilantro, chopped
- Lime juice
- Salt and pepper to taste

Instructions:

In a bowl, combine cooked quinoa, grilled chicken strips, diced mango, diced avocado, and finely chopped red onion.

Squeeze fresh lime juice over the ingredients.

Add chopped cilantro and season with salt and pepper.

Gently mix the ingredients until well combined.

Serve in bowls for a tropical and flavorful meal.

These recipes are easily customizable to suit your dietary requirements and tastes. Always consult with healthcare professionals or a registered dietitian for personalized dietary advice, especially when managing diverticulitis.

Soft Wraps and Sandwiches

Turkey and Avocado Wrap:

Ingredients:

- Soft whole-grain wrap
- Sliced turkey
- Mashed avocado
- Lettuce
- Light dressing (lemon vinaigrette or a yogurt-based dressing)

Instructions:

Lay the whole-grain wrap on a flat surface.

Layer sliced turkey, mashed avocado, and lettuce evenly across the wrap.

Drizzle with a light dressing of your choice.

Roll the wrap tightly, securing the filling inside.

Slice in half diagonally for serving.

Hummus and Vegetable Wrap:

Ingredients:

- Soft whole-grain wrap

- Hummus

- Roasted or raw vegetables (bell peppers, cucumbers, cherry tomatoes)

- Fresh spinach leaves

Instructions:

Spread a generous layer of hummus onto the whole-grain wrap.

Arrange the roasted or raw vegetables and fresh spinach leaves evenly.

Roll the wrap tightly, keeping the filling secure.

Slice into smaller portions for serving.

Avocado Chickpea Salad Wrap:

Ingredients:

- Soft wrap (whole-grain or spinach)

- Mashed avocado

- Chickpeas (canned, drained, and rinsed)

- Cherry tomatoes, halved

- Cilantro, chopped

- Salt and pepper to taste

Instructions:

Mash the avocado and spread it evenly onto the soft wrap.

In a bowl, mix chickpeas, halved cherry tomatoes, and chopped cilantro.

Season the chickpea mixture with salt and pepper.

Spoon the chickpea mixture onto the avocado-covered wrap.

Roll the wrap tightly, ensuring the filling is well-contained.

Slice into portions and serve.

Tuna Salad Spinach Wrap:

Ingredients:

- Soft spinach wrap
- Canned tuna, drained
- Mayonnaise
- Celery, finely chopped
- Shredded carrots
- Salt and pepper to taste

Instructions:

In a bowl, mix canned tuna, mayonnaise, finely chopped celery, shredded carrots, salt, and pepper.

Lay out the soft spinach wrap.

Spread the tuna salad mixture evenly on the wrap.

Roll the wrap tightly and slice it into portions for serving.

Mango Chicken Lettuce Wraps:

Ingredients:

- Soft lettuce leaves
- Grilled chicken, shredded
- Diced mango
- Mango salsa (tomatoes, red onion, cilantro, lime juice)
- Salt and pepper to taste

Instructions:

Mix the grilled chicken with diced mango in a bowl.

In a separate bowl, prepare mango salsa by combining tomatoes, red onion, cilantro, and lime juice.

Lay out soft lettuce leaves on a flat surface.

Spoon the chicken and mango mixture onto each lettuce leaf.

Top with mango salsa, and season with salt and pepper.

Serve the lettuce wraps with the filling.

Mushroom and Spinach Quesadilla:

Ingredients:

- Soft-flour tortilla
- Sliced mushrooms
- Fresh spinach leaves
- Shredded cheese (cheddar or Monterey Jack)
- Olive oil

Instructions:

In a pan, sauté sliced mushrooms in olive oil until cooked.

Place a soft-flour tortilla in the pan.

On one half of the tortilla, distribute shredded cheese.

Add sautéed mushrooms and fresh spinach leaves on top of the cheese.

Fold the tortilla in half, creating a quesadilla.

Cook until both sides of the tortilla are golden brown and the cheese has melted.

Slice into wedges and serve.

Feel free to experiment with these recipes, adjusting ingredients based on your preferences and dietary needs.

DINNER CREATIONS

Baked Fish with Herbs

Recipes for Baked Fish with Herbs Please

Simple and delicious recipe for Baked Fish with Herbs:

Baked Herb-Crusted Fish

Ingredients:

- 4 white fish fillets (such as tilapia or cod)

- 2 tablespoons olive oil

- 2 tablespoons fresh parsley, chopped

- 1 tablespoon fresh dill, chopped

- 1 tablespoon fresh thyme leaves

- 1 tablespoon fresh lemon juice

- 2 cloves garlic, minced

- Salt and pepper to taste

- Lemon wedges for serving

Instructions:

Preheat the Oven:

- Preheat your oven to 375°F (190°C).

Prepare the Fish:

- Using paper towels, pat dry the salmon fillets.

- Place the fillets on a baking sheet lined with parchment paper.

Herb Mixture:

- In a small bowl, mix together the olive oil, chopped parsley, dill, thyme, minced garlic, and lemon juice.

- Season the mixture with salt and pepper according to your taste.

Coat the Fish:

- Brush the herb mixture over the fish fillets, making sure to coat them evenly on both sides.

Bake:

- Place the baking sheet in the preheated oven.

- Bake for about 15-20 minutes or until the fish is cooked through and flakes easily with a fork.

Serve:

- Carefully transfer the baked fish fillets to serving plates.

- Garnish with additional fresh herbs if desired.

- Serve with lemon wedges on the side for a burst of citrus flavor.

Enjoy:

- Enjoy your delicious and herb-infused baked fish.

This baked fish recipe is not only flavorful but also a healthy option. Feel free to adjust the herb quantities based on your preferences, and consider serving it with a side of steamed vegetables or a light salad for a well-balanced meal.

Recipes for Steamed Vegetables with Lean Proteins.

Steamed Vegetables with Lemon Garlic Chicken

Ingredients:

- 2 boneless, skinless chicken breasts

- 2 tablespoons olive oil

- 3 cloves garlic, minced

- 1 teaspoon lemon zest

- 2 tablespoons lemon juice

- 1 teaspoon dried oregano

- Salt and pepper to taste

For the Steamed Vegetables:

- 2 cups broccoli florets

- 1 cup sliced carrots

- 1 cup snap peas, trimmed

- 1 red bell pepper, sliced

- 1 tablespoon olive oil

- Salt and pepper to taste

- Fresh parsley for garnish (optional)

Instructions:

Prepare the Chicken:

Recipes for One-Pot Meals for Easy Cleanup

Recipe for a One-Pot Chicken and Vegetable Skillet for easy cleanup:

One-Pot Chicken and Vegetable Skillet

Ingredients:

•   One pound of bite-sized pieces of boneless, skinless chicken breasts

•   2 tablespoons olive oil

•   1 onion, diced

•   2 bell peppers (any color), sliced

•   2 carrots, sliced

•   1 zucchini, sliced

•   2 cloves garlic, minced

•   1 teaspoon dried thyme

•   1 teaspoon dried rosemary

•   1 teaspoon paprika

•   Salt and pepper to taste

•   1 cup quinoa or rice

- 2 cups chicken broth

- Fresh parsley for garnish (optional)

Instructions:

Cook Chicken:

- Heat olive oil in a large skillet over medium-high heat.

- Add the chicken pieces and cook until browned on all sides. Take out of the skillet and place aside.

Sauté Vegetables:

- In the same skillet, add a bit more olive oil if needed.

- Sauté the diced onion, sliced bell peppers, carrots, and zucchini until the vegetables are slightly tender.

Season:

- Add minced garlic, dried thyme, dried rosemary, paprika, salt, and pepper to the vegetables. Stir well to coat.

Add Grains:

- Pour in quinoa or rice and stir to combine with the vegetables.

Combine with Chicken:

- Return the cooked chicken to the skillet and mix everything.

Pour Broth:

- Pour chicken broth into the skillet. Bring to a simmer.

Simmer and Cook:

- Reduce the heat to low, cover the skillet, and let it simmer until the grains are cooked and the chicken is cooked through, about 15-20 minutes.

Garnish and Serve:

- Once cooked, fluff the mixture with a fork.

- Garnish with fresh parsley if desired.

- Serve directly from the skillet.

This one-pot meal combines lean protein, colorful vegetables, and grains in a flavorful dish. To suit your tastes, change the seasonings and vegetables.

Yogurt Parfaits

A simple and delicious recipe for Yogurt Parfaits:

Berry and Granola Yogurt Parfait

Ingredients:

• Two cups Greek yogurt or any other yogurt of your choice

• 1/2 cup of granola

• 1 cup of mixed berries (strawberries, blueberries, and raspberries)

• 2 tablespoons of optional honey or maple syrup• Fresh mint leaves for garnish (optional)

Instructions:

Prepare the Yogurt:

- In a bowl, layer the bottom with a portion of Greek yogurt.

Add Mixed Berries:

- Add a layer of mixed berries on top of the yogurt.

Sprinkle Granola:

- Sprinkle a layer of granola over the berries.

Repeat Layers:

- Repeat the layers until the serving glass or bowl is filled, finishing with a layer of berries on top.

Drizzle with Honey or Maple Syrup (Optional):

- If desired, drizzle honey or maple syrup over the top for added sweetness.

Garnish with Mint (Optional):

- Garnish with fresh mint leaves for a burst of freshness.

Serve Immediately:

- Serve the yogurt parfait immediately for a delightful and nutritious breakfast or snack.

Feel free to customize your yogurt parfait with different fruits, nuts, or seeds based on your preferences. Yogurt parfaits are not only tasty but also versatile, providing a balance of protein, fiber, and natural sweetness. Enjoy this quick and healthy treat.

Fresh Fruit Snacks

Refreshing and easy recipe for Fresh Fruit Snacks:

Fresh Fruit Skewers with Honey-Lime Dip

Ingredients:

For Fruit Skewers:

- Assorted fresh fruits (such as strawberries, pineapple chunks, grapes, and melon balls)

- Wooden skewers

For Honey-Lime Dip:

- 1/4 cup honey

- Zest of one lime

- 2 tablespoons lime juice

- Fresh mint leaves for garnish (optional)

Instructions:

Prepare the Fruit:

- Wash and prepare the fresh fruits. If using larger fruits like melon, cut them into bite-sized chunks.

Skewer the Fruits:

- Thread the assorted fruits onto the wooden skewers, creating colorful and enticing fruit skewers.

Make the Honey-Lime Dip:

- In a small bowl, mix together honey, lime zest, and lime juice. Stir until well combined.

Serve:

- Arrange the fruit skewers on a platter.

- Drizzle the honey-lime dip over the skewers or serve it on the side as a dipping sauce.

Garnish (Optional):

- Garnish with fresh mint leaves for added flavor and a touch of greenery.

Enjoy:

- Serve these fresh fruit skewers with honey-lime dip as a healthy and vibrant snack.

This simple and colorful fruit snack is not only visually appealing but also a delightful way to enjoy the natural sweetness of fresh fruits. It's perfect for gatherings, parties, or as a refreshing treat on a hot day. Feel free to mix and match fruits based on your preferences.

Berry Compote with Greek Yogurt

Delightful recipe for Berry Compote with Greek Yogurt:

Berry Compote with Greek Yogurt

Ingredients:

For Berry Compote:

- 2 cups mixed berries (strawberries, blueberries, raspberries)

- 2 tablespoons honey or maple syrup

- 1 tablespoon lemon juice

- Zest of one lemon

- 1 teaspoon vanilla extract

For Serving:

- 2 cups Greek yogurt

- Fresh mint leaves for garnish (optional)

Instructions:

Prepare the Berries:

- Wash and hull the strawberries. If using larger berries, you can slice them for a uniform texture.

Cook the Berry Compote:

- In a saucepan, combine the mixed berries, honey or maple syrup, lemon juice, lemon zest, and vanilla extract.

- Heat over medium heat, stirring occasionally, until the berries release their juices and the mixture thickens slightly (about 8-10 minutes).

Mash or Keep Whole (Optional):

- If you prefer a smoother compote, you can use a potato masher to gently mash some of the berries. If you like it chunky, leave the berries whole.

Cool:

- Allow the berry compote to cool for a few minutes.

Assemble:

- Spoon a generous portion of Greek yogurt into serving bowls or glasses.

Top with Berry Compote:

- Spoon the warm or cooled berry compote over the Greek yogurt.

Garnish (Optional):

- Garnish with fresh mint leaves for a burst of freshness.

Serve:

- Serve immediately and enjoy this delicious Berry Compote with Greek Yogurt.

This delightful berry compote with creamy Greek yogurt is a perfect balance of sweetness and tanginess. It can be enjoyed as a healthy breakfast, a satisfying snack, or a light dessert. Feel free to customize the recipe with your favorite berries and adjust the sweetness according to your taste preferences.

Baked Apples with Cinnamon

Simple and comforting recipe for Baked Apples with Cinnamon:

Baked Apples with Cinnamon

Ingredients:

- 4 medium-sized apples (such as Granny Smith or Honeycrisp)

- 2 tablespoons unsalted butter, melted

- 1/4 cup brown sugar

- 1 teaspoon ground cinnamon

- 1/4 cup chopped nuts (pecans or walnuts), optional

- Vanilla ice cream or whipped cream for serving (optional)

Instructions:

Preheat the Oven:

- Preheat your oven to 375°F (190°C).

Prepare the Apples:

Wash and core the apples, leaving the
bottom intact to form a well for the filling.
You can use an apple corer or a small knife.

Mix the Filling:

- In a small bowl, mix together melted
  butter, brown sugar, and ground
  cinnamon until well combined.

Fill the Apples:

- Place the cored apples in a baking dish.

- Spoon the cinnamon-sugar mixture into the well
  of each apple.

Add Nuts (Optional):

- If using nuts, sprinkle chopped nuts over the top
  of each filled apple.

Bake:

- Bake the apples in the preheated oven for about
  25-30 minutes or until the apples are tender but
  not mushy.

Baste with Juices:

- Occasionally, spoon some of the juices from the baking dish over the apples while they bake for added flavor.

Serve:

Remove the baked apples from the oven.

Serve them warm, optionally topped with a scoop of vanilla ice cream or a dollop of whipped cream.

Enjoy:

- Enjoy the comforting aroma and delicious taste of baked apples with cinnamon.

This baked apple with cinnamon recipe is a simple and delightful dessert, perfect for a cozy evening. The combination of warm, tender apples with sweet cinnamon is both comforting and satisfying. Feel free to customize by adding your favorite nuts or adjusting the sweetness to your liking.

Low-Fiber Treats in Moderation

Recipe for a low-fiber treat that can be enjoyed in moderation:

Lemon Cheesecake Bites

Ingredients:

For the Crust:

- 1 cup finely ground graham cracker crumbs (choose a low-fiber option if available)

- 4 tablespoons unsalted butter, melted

- 2 tablespoons sugar

For the Cheesecake Filling:

- 8 ounces cream cheese, softened

- 1/2 cup sugar

- 1 teaspoon vanilla extract

- Zest of one lemon

- 2 tablespoons fresh lemon juice

- 2 large eggs

For Garnish (Optional):

- Whipped cream

- Fresh berries

- Mint leaves

Instructions:

Preheat the Oven:

- Preheat your oven to 325°F (163°C).

Prepare the Crust:

- In a bowl, combine the graham cracker crumbs, melted butter, and sugar.

- Press the mixture firmly into the bottom of a lined or greased mini muffin tin to create a crust.

- **Make the Cheesecake Filling:**

- In a separate bowl, beat the cream cheese until smooth.

- Add sugar, vanilla extract, lemon zest, and lemon juice. Mix until well combined.

- One egg at a time, adding and beating thoroughly after each addition.

Fill the Muffin Cups:

- Spoon the cheesecake filling into the prepared crust in each mini muffin cup.

Bake:

- Bake in the preheated oven for about 15-20 minutes or until the cheesecake is set.

Cool:

- Allow the cheesecake bites to cool in the muffin tin for a few minutes before transferring them to a wire rack to cool completely.

Chill:

- Place the cheesecake bites in the refrigerator and chill for at least 2 hours or until firm.

Garnish (Optional):

- If desired, garnish with a dollop of whipped cream, fresh berries, or mint leaves before serving.

Enjoy in Moderation:

- These lemon cheesecake bites are a delightful low-fiber treat that can be enjoyed in moderation.

These mini lemon cheesecake bites provide a burst of citrus flavor and a creamy texture, making them a delicious and satisfying low-fiber treat. Always remember to enjoy such treats in moderation and consult with healthcare professionals or a registered dietitian for personalized dietary advice, especially if managing specific health conditions.

MEAL PLANNING AND PREPARATION

Weekly Sample Meal Plans

Sample a weekly meal plan that incorporates a variety of nutrients while considering a balanced diet. Remember to adapt portions and ingredients based on personal preferences, dietary restrictions, and health goals.

Monday:

- Breakfast: Greek yogurt parfait with mixed berries and granola.

- Lunch: consists of grilled chicken salad dressed with balsamic vinaigrette, cucumber, cherry tomatoes, and mixed greens.

- Dinner: Baked salmon with lemon and herbs, quinoa, and steamed broccoli.

Tuesday:

- Breakfast: Whole grain toast with avocado and poached eggs.

- Lunch: Whole-grain crackers served alongside lentil soup.

- Dinner: Stir-fried tofu with colorful vegetables (bell peppers, broccoli, carrots) and brown rice.

Wednesday:

- Breakfast: Smoothie with spinach, banana, almond milk, and protein powder.

- Lunch: Quinoa salad with chickpeas, cherry tomatoes, cucumber, feta cheese, and a lemon-tahini dressing.

- Dinner: Grilled shrimp skewers, sweet potato wedges, and a side of asparagus.

Thursday:

- Breakfast: Oatmeal with sliced strawberries, almonds, and a drizzle of honey.

- Lunch: Turkey and avocado wrap with whole-grain tortilla.

- Dinner: Spaghetti squash with marinara sauce, lean ground turkey, and a side of mixed green salad.

Friday:

- **Breakfast:** Pineapple chunks combined with cottage cheese and chia seeds.

- **Lunch:** Quinoa-stuffed bell peppers with black beans, corn, and salsa.

- **Dinner:** Grilled chicken breast, roasted Brussels sprouts, and sweet potato mash.

Saturday:

- Breakfast: Whole grain pancakes with fresh blueberries and a dollop of Greek yogurt.

- Lunch: Caesar salad with grilled chicken, cherry tomatoes, croutons, and Caesar dressing.

- Dinner: Baked cod fillets with lemon-caper sauce, quinoa, and steamed green beans.

Sunday:

- **Breakfast:** Veggie omelet with spinach, tomatoes, bell peppers, and feta cheese.

- **Lunch:** Lentil, vegetable curry with brown rice.

- **Dinner:** Beef stir-fry with broccoli, snow peas, and carrots served over jasmine rice.

- **Snacks** (as needed throughout the week):

- Fresh fruit (e.g., apple slices, grapes)

* Raw veggies with hummus

Nuts or seeds

* Greek yogurt topped with a honey drizzle

Never forget to remain hydrated during the day by consuming lots of water. Adjust the meal plan to fit your dietary needs and preferences, and consider consulting with a registered dietitian for personalized advice.

Tips for Batch Cooking

Batch cooking is a time-saving and efficient way to prepare meals in advance. Tips for successful batch cooking:

Plan Your Menu:

* Start by planning a menu for the week. Choose recipes that are suitable for batch cooking and can be easily stored and reheated.

Choose Freezable Recipes:

- Opt for recipes that freeze well, such as casseroles, soups, stews, and sauces. These dishes often retain their flavor and texture when reheated.

Invest in Quality Storage Containers:

- Use a variety of airtight containers to store different types of dishes. Consider using freezer-safe containers to maintain food quality.

Label and Date Containers:

- Put the dish's name and preparation date on the label of each container. This guarantees that you utilize older things first and helps you keep track of freshness.

Prep Ingredients in Batches:

- Streamline the cooking process by chopping, slicing, and prepping ingredients in batches.

This makes it easier to assemble multiple meals quickly.

Use the Right Cooking Tools:

- Invest in kitchen tools that make batch cooking more efficient, such as a large slow cooker, instant pot, or sheet pans for roasting.

Cook in Bulk:

- Prepare larger quantities of staple ingredients like rice, quinoa, or roasted vegetables. These can be used as a base for different meals throughout the week.

Portion Control:

- Portion your meals into individual servings before freezing. This makes it easy to thaw and reheat exactly what you need.

Rotate Ingredients:

- Incorporate ingredients that can be used in multiple dishes. For example, roast a large batch of vegetables and use them in salads, wraps, or as side dishes.

Schedule Batch Cooking Sessions:

- Dedicate specific days or times during the week for batch cooking. This helps create a routine and ensures you always have a variety of meals on hand.

Avoid Overcooking:

- Be mindful of the cooking time, especially when batch cooking proteins. Overcooked meats can become dry when reheated.

Try One-Pot Meals:

- Simplify cleanup by preparing one-pot meals. These often involve less mess and fewer dishes to wash.

Consider a Meal Prep Day:

- Designate a day for meal prep where you can focus on batch cooking and assembling meals for the upcoming week.

Stay Organized:

- Keep a running inventory of what you have in your freezer. Regularly check and rotate items to use older ones first.

Experiment with Recipe Variations:

- Use your batch-cooked ingredients in different ways to avoid monotony. For instance, shredded chicken can be used in sandwiches, salads, or wraps.

Batch cooking can save time, money, and reduce stress during busy weeks. With a bit of planning and organization, you can enjoy the convenience of having homemade meals readily available.

Grocery Shopping for Diverticulitis-Friendly Ingredients

When shopping for diverticulitis-friendly ingredients, it's important to focus on foods that are gentle on the digestive system and lower in fiber.

Guide for grocery shopping with diverticulitis in mind:

Fresh Produce:

1. **Leafy Greens:**

   Opt for low-fiber greens such as spinach, iceberg lettuce, and peeled cucumbers.

2. **Cooked Vegetables:**

   Choose well-cooked and peeled vegetables like carrots, zucchini, and green beans.

3. **Fruits:**

   Select ripe and peeled fruits like bananas, melons, and peeled apples.

4. **Berries:**

Enjoy softer berries like blueberries and raspberries in moderation.

5. **Avocado:**

Avocado is generally well-tolerated and provides healthy fats.

Proteins:

6. **Lean Meats:**

Choose lean proteins like skinless poultry, fish, and lean cuts of beef or pork.

7. **Eggs:**

Eggs are a versatile and low-fiber protein option.

8. **Tofu:**

Tofu can be a good plant-based protein source.

Grains:

9. White Rice:

Opt for white rice instead of brown rice for lower fiber content.

10. White Bread and Pasta:

Choose white bread and pasta made from refined grains for lower fiber content.

Dairy and Alternatives:

11. Low-Fat Dairy:

Select low-fat or lactose-free dairy products like yogurt and milk.

12. Lactose-Free Milk:

If lactose intolerant, consider lactose-free milk or alternative milk options like almond or rice milk.

Canned and Cooked Foods:

13. Canned Vegetables and Fruits:

Choose canned fruits and vegetables that are softer and well-cooked.

14. Canned Fish:

Opt for canned fish like tuna or salmon for convenient protein.

Snacks:

15. Nut Butter:

Peanut butter or almond butter can be a good source of protein.

16. Low-Fiber Crackers:

Choose crackers made from refined flour with lower fiber content.

Beverages:

17. Herbal Teas:

Enjoy soothing herbal teas like peppermint or chamomile.

18. Infused Water:

Stay hydrated with infused water using fruits like lemon or cucumber.

Cooking Oils:

19. Olive Oil:

Use olive oil for cooking or dressing as it is a healthier fat option.

Sweeteners:

20. Honey or Maple Syrup:

Use natural sweeteners like honey or maple syrup in moderation.

Supplements:

21. Fiber Supplements:

If advised by a healthcare professional, consider soluble fiber supplements.

Prepackaged Meals:

22. Low-Fiber Soups:

Choose low-fiber soups, avoiding those with added seeds or tough vegetables.

Considerations:

23. Read Labels:

Check food labels to ensure low fiber content and avoid foods with seeds or tough skins.

24. Hydration:

Drink lots of water throughout the day to be well-hydrated.

2.5 Moderation:

Enjoy a variety of foods in moderation to maintain a balanced diet.

Always consult with a healthcare professional or a registered dietitian for personalized advice based on your specific health needs and dietary requirements. Adjust your choices based on your tolerance and preferences while managing diverticulitis.

CONCLUSION

Diverticulitis may be controlled with diet, but doing so requires planning and balance. "The Simple Diverticulitis Cookbook: 2024 Edition" is a useful tool that offers recipes together with advice on how to choose foods with awareness.

It's important to comprehend the nature of diverticulitis. The inflammation of tiny pouches (diverticula) in the digestive tract, which frequently develops in the colon, is known as diverticulitis. For the sake of digestive health, dietary fiber is typically recommended; but, during flare-ups, people with diverticulitis may benefit from a low-fiber or modified-fiber diet. This cookbook has a strong emphasis on dishes that are easy on the digestive system in an effort to reduce discomfort and promote general well-being.

Essential issues covered in the cookbook's table of contents include the role that nutrition plays in treating symptoms, the benefits of high-fiber foods for digestive health, explanations of low-residue diets, items to avoid, and substitutes. It also explores useful topics like portion control, gentle cooking methods, suggested tools and equipment, and even recipes for infused water and smoothies high in fiber.

A diverticulitis-friendly diet is supported by the sample dishes that are offered; they include Baked Fish with Herbs, Steamed Vegetables with Lean Proteins, and Berry Compote with Greek Yogurt. These recipes put an emphasis on using foods that are light on the stomach while yet producing tasty and fulfilling meals.

Batch cooking is a useful approach for successful deployment. Choosing recipes that can be frozen, organizing weekly dinners, and purchasing high-quality storage containers are all crucial components of batch cooking success. This method guarantees a consistent supply of diverticulitis-friendly foods throughout the week in addition to saving time.

When shopping for groceries, choose fresh fruit, lean meats, whole grains, dairy products or substitutes, and snacks that are compatible with diverticulitis. The focus is on selecting foods that are simple to digest, including refined grains, low-fiber fruits, and lean meats.

It's critical to maintain flexibility when controlling diverticulitis. Since everyone reacts to food differently, it's important to be aware of one's own tolerance levels and seek medical advice from qualified dietitians or other specialists.

By adopting a diverticulitis-friendly lifestyle, a comprehensive strategy to promote digestive health and general well-being may be created by combining a well-planned cookbook, thoughtful grocery shopping, smart batch cooking, and constant awareness of individual nutritional needs.

Recap of Diverticulitis Dietary Strategies

Let's recap the dietary strategies for managing diverticulitis:

Understanding Diverticulitis:

- Diverticulitis involves inflammation of small pouches (diverticula) in the digestive tract, primarily in the colon.

- During flare-ups, a low-fiber or modified-fiber diet may be recommended to minimize discomfort.

Importance of Diet in Managing Symptoms:

- Diet plays a crucial role in managing diverticulitis symptoms.

- Balancing fiber intake and choosing easily digestible foods can help alleviate symptoms.

High-Fiber Foods for Digestive Health:

- While diverticulitis may require a low-fiber approach during flare-ups, incorporating high-fiber foods during remission is generally beneficial.

- High-fiber foods include fruits, vegetables, whole grains, and legumes.

Low-Residue Diet Explained:

- A low-residue diet limits the intake of foods that leave undigested remnants in the colon, reducing the workload on the digestive system.

- Cooked and peeled vegetables, well-cooked grains, and lean proteins are often included in a low-residue diet.

Foods to Avoid and Alternatives:

- Foods with seeds, nuts, and tough skins should be avoided during diverticulitis flare-ups.

- Opt for alternatives like seedless fruits, well-cooked vegetables, and tender meats.

Gentle Cooking Techniques:

- Gentle cooking techniques, such as baking, steaming, or poaching, help maintain the integrity of ingredients while making them easier to digest.

Recommended Utensils and Equipment:

- Using appropriate utensils and equipment, like non-stick pans or slow cookers, can aid in preparing easily digestible meals.

Portion Control:

- Controlling portion sizes is essential to avoid overloading the digestive system.

- Smaller, more frequent meals may be preferable to larger, infrequent ones.

Fiber-Rich Smoothies:

- Fiber-rich smoothies can be a nutritious and easy-to-digest option, incorporating ingredients like peeled fruits, yogurt, and soluble fiber sources.

Infused Water Recipes:

- Staying hydrated is crucial. Infused water with gentle flavors like cucumber or lemon can be a refreshing alternative.

Herbal Teas for Soothing the Digestive Tract:

- Herbal teas like peppermint or chamomile can have soothing effects on the digestive tract.

Oatmeal Variations:

- Oatmeal, when prepared with well-cooked oats and gentle toppings, can be a comforting and low-residue breakfast option.

Managing diverticulitis involves a nuanced approach to diet, considering individual tolerance levels and adapting to both flare-ups and remission periods. Incorporating these dietary strategies can help promote digestive health and overall well-being. Always consult with healthcare professionals or a registered dietitian for personalized advice based on individual health needs.

Encouragement for Long-Term Wellness

Embarking on a journey toward long-term wellness, especially when managing a condition like diverticulitis, requires commitment and resilience. Here's some encouragement for your path to lasting well-being:

Consistency is Key:

- Wellness is not about perfection but about consistency. Small, sustainable changes in your diet and lifestyle over time can lead to significant improvements.

Celebrate Progress, Big or Small:

- Take a moment to celebrate every step forward, whether it's trying a new diverticulitis-friendly recipe, successfully completing a gentle workout, or making mindful choices at the grocery store.

Listen to Your Body:

- Pay attention to how your body responds to different foods and activities. Your body is unique, and understanding its signals is a powerful tool on your wellness journey.

Embrace Adaptability:

- Wellness is a dynamic process. Be open to adjusting your strategies as needed, based on your evolving needs and insights about what works best for you.

Self-Care is Vital:

- Prioritize self-care in your routine. Whether it's taking a moment for deep breathing, enjoying a peaceful walk, or indulging in a favorite hobby, self-care nourishes both your body and mind.

Build a Support System:

- Surround yourself with a supportive network—friends, family, healthcare professionals, or a wellness community. Having a support system can provide encouragement, share experiences, and offer valuable insights.

Mindfulness Matters:

- Incorporate mindfulness into your daily life. Whether it's practicing mindful eating, engaging in meditation, or simply being present in the moment, mindfulness can enhance your overall sense of well-being.

Focus on What You Can Control:

- While certain aspects of health may be beyond your control, focus on the choices you can make daily. Small, positive decisions accumulate over time and contribute to your long-term wellness.

Educate Yourself:

- Knowledge is empowering. Continue to educate yourself about diverticulitis, nutrition, and holistic well-being. The more informed you are, the better equipped you'll be to make choices aligned with your health goals.

Patience and Perseverance:

- Wellness is a journey, not a destination. Be patient with yourself, and understand that progress may come gradually. Perseverance in the face of challenges is a testament to your commitment to long-term health.

Celebrate Non-Scale Victories:

- Not all victories are measured on a scale. Celebrate improvements in energy levels, better digestion, or increased resilience. These non-scale victories are significant indicators of your overall health.

Prioritize Joy:

- Infuse joy into your wellness journey. Find activities that bring you happiness and make them a regular part of your routine. Joy is a powerful motivator and contributor to long-term well-being.

Remember, your journey towards long-term wellness is uniquely yours. Each positive choice, no matter how small, is a step in the right direction. Embrace the process; be kind to yourself, and savor the rewards of a life lived with well-being in mind. You've got this!

www.ingramcontent.com/pod-product-compliance
Lightning Source LLC
Chambersburg PA
CBHW050819260726

48660CB00004B/1521